A GENERAL PRACTITIONER,
HIS PATIENTS

CW01081763

A GENERAL PRACTITIONER, HIS PATIENTS AND THEIR FEELINGS

Exploring the Emotions
Behind Physical Symptoms

SOTIRIS ZALIDIS

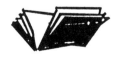

FREE ASSOCIATION BOOKS / LONDON / NEW YORK

First published in 2001 by
FREE ASSOCIATION BOOKS
57 Warren Street, London W1T 5NR

www.fa-b.com

Copyright © Sotiris Zalidis 2001

The right of Sotiris Zalidis to be identified as the author of this work has
been asserted by him in accordance with the Copyright, Designs and
Patents Act 1988.

A CIP catalogue record for this book is available from the British Library

ISBN 1 85343 527 9 pbk

10 09 08 07 06 05 04 03 02 01
10 9   8   7   6   5   4   3   2   1

Designed and produced for Free Association Books by
Chase Publishing Services, Fortescue, Sidmouth EX10 9QG
Printed in the European Union by Antony Rowe Ltd, Chippenham, England

CONTENTS

To Dr Popi Zalidis whose example taught me that aristocracy of character is the only form of nobility that merits admiration.

ACKNOWLEDGEMENTS

Writing a book evokes many complex emotions and one among them is gratitude for all the help received in completing what was felt to be a huge task. Although I have to take full responsibility for the contents of the book, the clarity of the ideas and precision of language would be a lot less if it was not for the help of friends and colleagues. I would like to thank them in alphabetical order.

Dr Abe Brafman for reading the final version of the first section of chapter 10 and making important clarifications. Dr Alexis Brook for reading the second draft of Chapter 13 and making helpful comments and corrections. His research at the Well Street Surgery on the emotions behind eye disorders inspired that chapter. Trevor Brown, the editor of Free Association Books who believed I could write this book and urged me to do so. Dr Chris Griffiths for reading very carefully the second draft of Chapter 4 and for making corrections and important clarifications. He has been the clinical tutor supervising the research on herpes zoster on which this chapter is based. Tirril Harris for teaching me how to use the life events and difficulties schedule. Also for being enthusiastic about the herpes zoster project and inviting me to present my cases regularly to her consensus meetings. Professor Dick Joyce for his extraordinarily generous offer to edit the whole manuscript. He very tactfully made suggestions that improved the style of my prose.

Dr Julie Nye for being the only colleague to read part of the first draft and for making useful suggestions. My partners, Drs Paul Julian, Gabriella Tobias, Nick Hutt, Jo Hayman, Fiona Bernard and Cathy Highton, for supporting the research projects on hyperventilation, herpes zoster and psychosomatic eye conditions, on which chapters 4, 5 and 13 are based.

Hermione Pool for her helpful comments and advice on the first section of chapter 10. She was the Well Street Surgery practice nurse as well as counsellor when I treated the asthmatic patient referred to in that chapter. Dr Peter Shoenberg for sharing my interest in psychosomatic medicine and for introducing me to Professor Joyce. Also for all the stimulating conversations we have had over the years which helped shape my psychosomatic ideas. The psychosomatic workshop he runs at the Department of Psychotherapy at University College Hospital has provided a forum where some of the material that became Chapters 4, 5, 6 and 10 was presented for the first time. Professor Lesley Southgate for being interested in my approach and for inviting me to become a research associate at the department of general practice at St Bartholomew's Hospital. The purpose of this invitation was to write a proposal for a research project testing my ideas on the emotional setting within which herpes zoster erupts. Chapter 4 is based on the research that followed. Professor Graeme Taylor for writing the foreword to this book and allowing me to use the Toronto Alexithymia Scale. His books have been an education for me. Dr Peter White for discussing the herpes zoster project and suggesting that the life events and difficulties schedule would be the best way to measure stress.

Lynn and Katerina Zalidis for feeling proud that I was writing this book and always encouraging me to persevere with the project. Their positive emotions helped me tolerate my doubts about its value and gave me the strength to continue.

The following publications are quoted by permission.

M. Balint, *The Doctor, His Patient and the Illness* (Pitman Medical, 1957). By kind permission of Harcourt Publishers Ltd.

H. Krystal, *Integration and Self-Healing. Affect, Trauma, Alexithymia* (The Analytic Press, 1988). By kind permission of The Analytic Press.

J. Le Doux, *The Emotional Brain* (Weidenfeld and Nicolson, 1998). By kind permission of The Orion Publishing Group.

J. D. Lane and A. Storr, *Asthma: The Facts* (Oxford University Press, 1981). By kind permission of Oxford University Press.

W. I. Miller, *The Anatomy of Disgust* (Harvard University Press, 1997). By kind permission of Harvard University Press.

D. L. Nathanson, *Shame and Pride. Affect Sex and the Birth of the Self* (W. W. Norton & Co., 1992). By kind permission of W. W. Norton & Co.

W. F. Platt, *Conversation Repair. Case Studies in Doctor–Patient Communication* (Little, Brown & Co., 1995). By kind permission of Warner Books.

J. M. D. Stoller, *Observing the Erotic Imagination* (Yale University Press, 1985). By kind permission of Yale University Press.

G. J. Taylor, *Psychosomatic Medicine and Contemporary Psychoanalysis* (International Universities Press, 1987). By kind permission of International Universities Press.

D. W. Winnicott, 'The observation of infants in a set situation' in his *Through Paediatrics to Psycho-Analysis* (Hogarth Press, 1975). By kind permission of Mark Paterson and Associates.

AUTHOR'S NOTE

CONFIDENTIALITY

In this book I have taken great care to protect the identity of all patients by changing their names, occupations and nationalities. However, the one thing I could not change was the fact that every narrative is unique. I hope that by being true to the stories I am contributing to a debate that might help promote a humane medical attitude. Had I made up fictitious narratives to approximate the real ones my account would have lost much of its authenticity.

A COMMENT ABOUT THE 'HE' PRONOUN

The use of **he** as a pronoun for nouns embracing both genders is a simple, practical convention rooted in the beginnings of the English language ... it has no pejorative connotations; it is never incorrect.

(William Strunk Jr and E.B. White. *The Elements of Style* (3rd edn). New York: Macmillan, 1979, p. 60)

FOREWORD

Graeme J. Taylor, MD FRCPC MRCPsych
Professor of Psychiatry, University of Toronto

Emotions are a striking and omnipresent feature of human experience. Although they are rooted in biology and clearly discernible in the behaviour of many other animals, we know our emotions best through our subjective feelings. In any one day we may experience anger, fear, love, hate, joy, interest, shame, pride and disgust. And over the course of days or weeks, our moods also are influenced by emotional states; we may be elated, depressed, irritable or merely contented, sometimes for obvious reasons but often without knowing why. Emotions motivate and influence much of our behaviour; we may be compelled to run when we are afraid, can remain absorbed in a task when we experience interest, and may be moved to comfort friends when we feel their distress. And while powerful events generally evoke intense emotional responses, such as grief following the loss of a loved one, even minor slights can evoke furious rage that may lead to irrational behaviour.

In addition to their motivational effects, emotions communicate information to ourselves and others. Through an awareness of distinctive feelings, we are informed about our internal states and our responses to people and events in our external environment; through distinctive facial and vocal expressions, we communicate some of this information to others. Similarly, we gain knowledge of the emotional states of others from our perception and understanding of their non-verbal expressions. Although other mammals may have a rudimentary conscious appreciation of their emotional states, the more highly evolved neocortex and its associated capacity for symbolization and language in humans alters the way emotions are experienced, and also enables us to reflect upon our subjective feelings. As the neuroscientist Joseph Le Doux (1996) points out, 'feelings [are] different in a brain that can classify the world linguistically and categorize experience in words, than in a brain that cannot'.

People obviously vary in their capacity to be attuned to emotions in themselves and others, and in their ability to accurately describe emotional experience. In his theory of multiple intelligences, the educational psychologist Howard Gardner (1983) described two subtypes of personal intelligence

– *intrapersonal intelligence*, which he defined as the ability to access one's own feeling life and to use this information to understand and guide one's behaviour; and *interpersonal intelligence*. Within the fields of psychoanalysis and psychosomatic medicine, however, and for the last fifty years, clinicians have observed that certain patients have difficulty identifying and describing subjective feelings, and show an associated limited capacity for fantasy and imaginative play, presumably because their emotions are poorly represented mentally. Empirical research over the past decade has shown that these so-called *alexithymic* individuals experience their emotions largely as bodily sensations and impulses to action, and/or poorly differentiated unidimensional feelings. Confused and bewildered by their emotions, they cope poorly with stressful situations and seem particularly prone to eating disorders, substance use disorders and medically unexplained somatic symptoms (Taylor et al. 1997).

Other individuals, especially those with borderline personality features, appear at times to experience too much emotion. Although this emotion also is often poorly differentiated, it is used frequently by these individuals to coerce others, including physicians, into meeting their dependent needs. Many psychiatric patients experience too much or too little emotion. Those with bipolar disorders for example, experience an excess of the affect interest – excitement when they are hypomanic, and too little of this affect when they are depressed. The idea that excessive and unregulated levels of negative emotion can have adverse influences on physical health has been expressed by physicians and philosophers since ancient times. However, this view was not given much attention until the late eighteenth century when the eminent physician William Falconer published a book entitled *The Influence of the Passions upon Disorders of the Body*. It took another century and the emergence and influence of psychoanalysis before psychosomatic medicine became a respected discipline for studying the role of emotions in health and disease.

Human emotions and the benefits and problems associated with them are nowhere more evident than in the consulting room of the general practitioner. As Dr Sotiris Zalidis declares in the title of the second chapter of this remarkable book, 'general practice is the playing field of human emotions'. Through the many detailed case histories he provides throughout the book, Dr Zalidis sensitively transmits to the reader a powerful sense of the anxieties, anger, shame, sadness and hope experienced by his patients as they struggle with the suffering of illness in themselves or in their loved ones, and sometimes also with the loneliness of facing death. This is a privileged involvement in other people's lives which may be granted primarily to the general practitioner or to a close friend, rabbi or clergyman who provides counsel. But the author draws us even further into sampling the emotional drama that so often emerges in the doctor–patient encounter, as he also openly shares with us his own emotional responses to his patients and their suffering, and describes how he uses these reactions to gain a greater understanding of their psychological states. In so doing he captures the flavour of much contemporary psychoanalytic thinking about intersubjectivity and countertransference, as well as the multifaceted ways in which bodily experiences enter into the relational matrix. In his approach to patients, Dr Zalidis departs from the prevailing biomedical model of disease and practises a holistic medicine in which he incorporates principles and ideas propounded by the American psychosomaticists, Engel and Schmale, as well as those contributed by British psychoanalysts, in particular Balint and Winnicott. By studying the life setting in which illness develops, Engel and Schmale (1967; Schmale 1972) discovered that the onset or exacerbation of disease is often triggered by intense feelings of helplessness and hopelessness in response to an important loss. Sometimes the memory of the loss has been repressed, but the unresolved affects may return with accompanying somatic sequelae, as in the clinical examples of anniversary reactions that are described in this book.

Like Balint, Engel discovered that often the most effective remedy for such patients is the empathic relationship established between the patient and the doctor. Dr Zalidis expands these observations by applying Winnicott's (1965) concept of the holding environment to the general practice setting, where the doctor's availability and affective attunement to the patient's verbal and non-verbal communications informs him when to intervene supportively to help alleviate the patient's fear of falling into a black hole of despair. This truly is the art of listening, whereby the doctor draws on his own emotional intelligence to employ affect as a sixth sense to discern the unarticulated mental state of the patient. Although the time constraints of a busy general practice obviously limit the full exploration of a patient's emotions, Dr Zalidis demonstrates how just a few carefully worded enquiries about the patient's fears can have therapeutic benefit. But when longer appointments can be scheduled, he shows also how a psychotherapeutically trained general practitioner can use more sophisticated techniques, including dream analysis and Winnicott's squiggle game, to explore powerful emotional states and thereby favourably influence the clinical course of illness or disease. Henry Krystal's (1988) important work on affect regression and its psychotherapeutic management is especially helpful for understanding and treating patients who present with functional somatic symptoms such as those associated with hyperventilation and panic attacks.

General practice is where most people first seek medical help and where they expect to encounter a humane doctor who respects their individuality. Nowadays, however, with the greater reliance on medical technology and the movement toward evidence-based medicine, there are risks that patient care will become increasingly dehumanised as physicians are encouraged to help reduce health costs by investigating and treating diseases and syndromes only, rather than the person as well as the disease. Dr Zalidis's emphasis on attending to patient's emotions, and the influence these have on bodily processes and bodily experience, underscores an observation made wisely by Balint (1965) over three decades ago, that 'more often than scientific medicine cares to admit, it is not with the part but the whole man that something has gone wrong'. Hopefully modern medicine, as it enters a new millennium, will embrace the exciting new and rapidly expanding understanding of emotion that is coming from neuroscience research (Le Doux 1996, Panksepp 1998), and thereby gain a greater appreciation of the centrality of emotions in human life and their importance in sickness and health.

REFERENCES

Balint, M. (1965) 'The doctor's therapeutic function'. *Lancet* 1:1177–80.

Engel, G. L. and Schmale, A. H. (1967). 'Psychoanalytic theory of somatic disorder: Conversion, specificity and the disease onset situation'. *Journal of the American Psychoanalytic Association* 15: 344–65.

Gardner, H. (1983). *Frames of Mind. The theory of multiple intelligences.* Basic Books, New York.

Krystal, H. (1988) *Integration and Self-healing: Affect, trauma, alexithymia.* Analytic Press, Hillsdale, NJ.

Le Doux, J. (1996) *The Emotional Brain.* Simon and Schuster, New York.

Panksepp, J. (1998) *Affective Neuroscience: The foundations of human and animal emotions.* Oxford University Press, New York.

Schmale, A. H. (1972) 'Giving up as a final common pathway to changes in health'. *Advances in Psychosomatic Medicine* 8: 21–40.

Taylor, G. J., Bagby, R. M. and Parker, J. D. A. (1997) *Disorders of Affect Regulation: Alexithymia in medical and psychiatric illness.* Cambridge University Press, Cambridge.

Winnicott, D. W. (1965) *The Maturational Processes and the Facilitating Environment.* Hogarth Press, London.

1 INTRODUCTION

> The patient to the doctors:
> Name me no name for my disease
> With uninforming breath;
> I tell you I am none of these
> But homesick unto death.
>   Witter Bynner, *Selected Poems.*

MY PROFESSIONAL DEVELOPMENT

This book is about the ideas I have found useful and the attitudes I have developed, in an effort to practise whole person medicine during my first thirteen years as a principal in general practice.

I first became interested in the whole person model when I was a student at the medical school of Athens in Greece. In 1974, one year after I graduated, I came to London in order to specialise in psychodynamic psychiatry.

As part of my training, I started personal analysis, but three years later, I revised my career plans and decided to pursue my earlier interest in psychosomatic medicine instead. As I realised that for this purpose I needed much more experience in general medicine than I already had, I worked in hospital medical posts for six years until I passed the examination for Membership of the Royal College of Physicians in 1982. At that point I began looking for a clinical setting which would allow me to integrate my psychiatric and medical experience. Discussions with Dr Rosalie Taylor, Dr Michael Courtenay and Dr Peter Shoenberg, were fundamental in convincing me that general practice was the setting I was looking for. All three were familiar with the pioneering work of Michael Balint and his collaborators in establishing the usefulness of applying psychodynamic ideas to general practice.

A year after completing my vocational training at Kentish Town Health Centre, during which I worked as a locum in a great variety of general practices, I was appointed partner at Well Street Surgery, a training group practice of doctors sympathetic to Balint's work. In December 1993 Mannie Sher, the course organising tutor of the British Association of Psychotherapists invited me to teach psychosomatic medicine at a course for counsellors in general practice. The four lectures I prepared for this purpose became the nucleus around which this book was written. However, my initial enthusiasm for the whole person model was soon tempered by the realisation that there is great resistance to it, not only among patients but also among doctors and even psychotherapists. There are a number of reasons why this may be so.

First, there is something comforting about the separation of body from mind which partly explains why the Cartesian split has endured for so long. This resistance against owning up to our unwanted emotional states and integrating their somatic with their cognitive components is deeply ingrained in British culture and encoded in the English language. Donald Winnicott has recognised the defensive function of this body/mind divide and has stated that the true illness in psychosomatic disorder is the persistence of a dissociation in the personality rather than the clinical state expressed in terms of somatic pathology (Winnicott 1964).

Second, whole person, or psychosomatic medicine, is essentially a practical discipline as well as a humbling one. The need for physical treatment of the body limits the scope for purely psychological interventions. Too much emphasis on the mind can be perceived by some patients as at best a dismissal of the reality of their suffering and at worst as a violation of their right for care, or as abandonment. To practise psychosomatic medicine one has to tolerate uncertainty about diagnosis and this is easier if the doctor has a proficient knowledge of medicine which allows him to consider and investigate alternative diagnoses.

Third, psychosomatic medicine, by introducing an added level of complexity, goes against our hunger for simplicity. Despite evidence that we live in a very complex world, we still desire simple and clear-cut rules and guidelines that will make everything easy by removing doubt and uncertainty. The psychosomatic approach involves an understanding of psychological, biological and sociological systems and their interaction and integration in each patient, whatever symptoms or disorder they may be suffering from.

Psychosomatic medicine reflects the fact that the human condition is multideterminate; it is not helpful to try to find a single cause for every symptom.

Finally, despite the growing recognition that emotional factors have a significant influence upon our health, there is not yet a consensus about the teaching of psychosomatic medicine in the United Kingdom. To complicate matters further, alternative or complementary approaches and oriental disciplines, such as acupuncture or Ayurvedic medicine use specific terminology to convey their holistic orientation.

Absence of a leading influence results in a multitude of conceptual frameworks that attempt to formulate body–mind interactions which inform a variety of clinical practices.

My own has been influenced greatly by the work of Michael Balint, Donald Winnicott and that of affect theorists exemplified by Henry Krystal and

Graeme Taylor, who have argued for an increasing emphasis on emotional development and emotional regulation within a psychodynamic framework.

Indeed, the title of the book pays homage to the work of Michael Balint, whose book *The Doctor, his Patient and the Illness* introduced psychodynamic thinking in general practice and asserted that whole person medicine is the province of the general practitioner. His own holistic approach was based on the notion of the 'basic fault', a term he used in a geological sense to mean an inherent weakness in the formation of personality, rather than in the sense of blame. He believed that the early months of a child's life, brought about an inevitable mismatch between individual needs and environmental care. This resulted in a constitutional vulnerability or 'basic fault' in the psyche/soma of the individual; the depth of the fault depended on the content of the mismatch and on individual temperament. The basic fault, according to Balint, predisposes the individual to problems which may be psychological and/or somatic and which tend to appear in times of stress.

Michael Balint and later Enid Balint began to lead training groups with general practitioners in the 1950s. This work resulted in the book *The Doctor, his Patient and the Illness*. Gradually, over the years, his ideas evolved and research groups under his guidance and that of his wife Enid, developed the 'Balint approach'. This was a move away from elaborate assessment and analytic interviews, to study the here and now relationships with the doctor. The doctor's increased understanding of the relationship with the patient, enables him to become more tolerant and more receptive to what the patient is saying, without necessarily attempting to challenge defences or make interpretations. The resulting improved relationship with the doctor can lead to a therapeutic change in the patient (Salinsky 1999).

Donald Winnicott, who was a paediatrician for many years before he became a psychoanalyst, studied the interaction between mother and baby and wrote in detail about what the ordinary devoted mother does naturally in order to prevent a mismatch between the needs of her baby and the caretaking environment. He emphasised the analogy between the activities of the ordinary 'good enough mother' who provides a 'facilitating environment' for the development of her baby's 'maturational processes' and the activities of the 'good enough doctor' who provides a supportive environment for the unfolding of the patient's innate tendency for 'integration' and 'self-healing'. His concept of 'holding' is particularly relevant for the work of general practitioners and is closely related to the capacity to tolerate emotions in reasonable comfort, to distinguish between different competing emotional states and to find the words to describe them accurately. A doctor who has had the experience of being held, either in personal analysis or within a Balint group, is better equipped to provide effective holding for his patients.

It is in this context that I have found the scientific language of affect theory very helpful in educating my ability to make finer and more appropriate discriminations between my personal feelings and with respect to reading the emotional signals of my patients. Although the science of emotions is still controversial, there is consensus among affect theory and contemporary psychoanalysis in considering emotions as primary motivating factors and multidimensional phenomena that are essential for communication and survival.

THE CHALLENGE OF GENERAL PRACTICE

Although there is evidence from general practice that longer consultations are of higher quality (Applefou, K. et al. 1998), doctors are often obliged to work faster and faster in order to accommodate the increasing number of patients who demand to be seen. It is gradually being acknowledged that a system of care that exhausts doctors and other health care professionals and makes them feel like hamsters on a treadmill is not sustainable (Smith, R. 2000).

One of the paradoxes of general practice is that although the relationship with some patients can extend over many years and the total time spent with them can add up to several hours, individual consultations in the surgery may last only a few minutes and are often conducted in a hurry. Our own practice manager has calculated that I have about 5,574 consultations a year. On a busy day I may have to see fifty patients and I may be interrupted several times during my consultations in order to deal with urgent requests to see patients who are sometimes too frightened or impatient to wait for a routine appointment. Sometimes the intensity of the work can be so great that it can activate negative emotions in me, not only because patients' negative emotions are catching, but also through the sheer volume and speed of work which can be greater than I can tolerate comfortably.

Expressions used by general practitioners to describe some aspects of their work, such as 'working on the coal face' or 'triage', convey the experience of being in the front line and working under fire in the day to day battle against the consequences of abuse, deprivation, disease and ignorance. The challenge in general practice is to do humane work whilst working at an inhuman pace.

Most patients come to the general practitioner when they need him in his administrative role, or when they feel generally unwell for any reason, or for a combination of the two. They come when they are worried about the significance of their symptoms or when they are annoyed with them. They hope that they will be met by a helpful attitude that will provide some relief from their distress or some magic that will get rid of it. The general practitioner, therefore, is at the receiving end of the patient's emotional communication from the moment the two meet. However, because affective experiences, more often than not, occur without an emotional label such as fear, sadness or impatience, it is possible for both doctor and patient to remain unaware of the presence of these affective states which may be very important in shaping the expectations of the patient. Of course, general practitioners have to be constantly vigilant and consider the possibility that the symptoms are due to a known disease. We reassure ourselves that we are not missing an important medical condition by doing the appropriate physical examination and ordering the relevant laboratory investigations, but we do not always find a medical explanation for the patient's symptoms. This does not mean that we can dismiss the patient. Being generalists we do not limit our help and understanding to medical problems alone but we are legitimately concerned with the whole gamut of human experience, and emotions are no exception. It is well known that emotions can manifest themselves with physical symptoms or maladaptive behaviours and, when they are not regulated, can also contribute to the disregulation of other biological systems, becoming a factor in the development of disease. Another paradox therefore is that although emotions are present in every consultation we tend to ignore them. We are skilled in performing intimate physical examinations, but we may feel awkward about examining the patient's feelings, which after all is an intimate examination, and rarely make the emotional communication explicit. During my working experience in general practice I have come to realise that unless I find the confidence to ask my patient what he is afraid may be wrong with him and put my finger on his feelings – so to speak – by examining them as calmly and objectively as I might any other part of his body, I might miss an important opportunity to target my reassurance specifically to his fears. Leaving the emotions in the darkness of the patient's unformulated thoughts and out of awareness, can only make them grow out of proportion and distort the doctor–patient relationship.

To be involved at the level of unexamined emotions can be harmful. If we fail to recognise and acknowledge our own feelings as well as the emotions of our patients we are at risk of acting them out by forgetfulness, by making mistakes, by being cruel to the patient or by neglecting our own needs. A survey published in 2000 by the Mental Health Foundation found that 44 per cent of the respondents experienced their general practitioner as unsympathetic and showing lack of understanding of their mental distress (Chada 2000). Doctors are not trained to make diagnoses of emotional states but to make diagnoses of medical diseases, and we feel most effective when we are given the pharmacological and physical means to fix them. In contrast, we repudiate the helplessness we may feel when we experience our own and our patients' intense affective states and we may feel guilty that we cannot be as effective in treating emotional pain, such as that of despair, as we are in treating the pain of a broken limb. We tend to underestimate, however, the relief some of our patients feel when we are interested enough to listen to their stories with sympathy and capable enough to accept and accurately recognise their feelings.

This book traces my effort to make good a deficiency in my medical training which did not include the teaching of emotions as a vital aspect of living physiology, the knowledge of which is necessary for understanding human beings (Zalidis 1991–99). This requires not only a knowledge of the contribution of the emotions to the formation of physical symptoms and predisposition to disease, but also the development of helpful attitudes towards oneself and the patient that make it safe to acknowledge and experience feelings that our upbringing and education have led us to consider shameful, dangerous and unacceptable.

This way of working is delicate and emotionally demanding. It needs to be nurtured, encouraged and facilitated by recognition and respect of the doctor's own needs and feelings. Illustrations of this need form one of the major themes of this book.

2 GENERAL PRACTICE IS THE PLAYING FIELD OF HUMAN EMOTIONS

Chorus: Did your offence perhaps go further than you have said?
Prometheus: Yes: I caused men no longer to foresee their death.
Chorus: What cure did you discover for their misery?
Prometheus: I planted firmly in their hearts blind hopefulness.
Aeschylus, *Prometheus Bound*.
(Penguin Classics. Translated by Philip Vellacott)

SEARCHING FOR A HUMANE MEDICAL ATTITUDE

Perhaps it is human nature that when we are looked after well, we take good care for granted, just as we take the air we breathe for granted. We do not become aware of our need for air until its absence makes us suffocate. So it is only when medical care fails our patients and their carers in some respect, and their hurt feelings compel them to tell us or write about their experiences, that we find out about the medical attitudes which they experience as inhuman.

In a moving account, the next of kin of Jeffrey, a consultant surgeon who died at the age of sixty-nine at home from acute myeloid leukaemia within five months from diagnosis, describes her experience of medical inhumanity in a letter to the *British Medical Journal* (anonymous contribution, 1994). The medical attitudes that she found most painful were an apparent lack of interest in Jeffrey's quality of life; lack of kindness, compassion and understanding of their feelings, and the team approach which has become a euphemism for lack of continuity.

Her description of the ward round after Jeffrey was admitted to hospital for chemotherapy has a familiar ring. Once each week, the medical team visited the wards. They could often be heard marching down the corridor before they entered smartly without knocking; the consultant first, followed deferentially by the team. The members of the team were constantly changing and it was impossible to keep up with who was who. They seemed hardly to look at the patient and appeared unmoved by his appearance, no matter how ghastly. After about four minutes, they all marched out of the room to visit the next patient.

As Jeffrey did not respond he was discharged home where his friend was condemned to observe Jeffrey's suffering and rapid physical deterioration without any emotional support from his doctors. Although the regular general practitioner, Dr K, had asked a few times about how Jeffrey was coping psychologically, at no time did he offer any help to make him comfortable. On Jeffrey's last day his breathing was noisy and he was distressed. His partner called the general practitioner, but Dr H – who was standing in for Dr K – arrived. Jeffrey wanted a tranquilliser for some relief of his distress, but Dr H was worried that it might depress Jeffrey's respiratory centre and offered methadone instead. Even at this late stage Jeffrey did not want methadone because he was afraid that it might kill him and he did not want to die. He insisted on a tranquilliser and Dr H left without prescribing anything. Later that day Jeffrey's own doctor was contacted and he agreed to administer the wished-for tranquilliser.

The patient died a few hours later. Jeffrey's partner felt that their physical and mental suffering was not understood and therefore they were not treated with kindness, even though from a technical point of view the chemotherapy was administered according to the latest scientific evidence and the treatment itself was part of a survey of the effects of cytotoxics on people over fifty years of age.

An important problem in treating sick people arises when medical personnel ignore how patients are reacting emotionally while their physical condition is being treated. Traditionally medicine has a very narrow view of health. Our training concentrates mainly on disease and ignores the patient's experience of disease which we can call illness. This inattention to the emotional reality of disease neglects a growing body of evidence that people's emotional states can sometimes play a significant role in their vulnerability to disease and in their response to treatment and recovery.

One of the most powerful demonstrations of the clinical power of emotional support was reported in groups for women with advanced metastatic breast cancer, at Stanford University Medical School. After the initial treatment, often including surgery, the cancers had returned and they were spreading. It was only a matter of time until the spreading cancer killed them. Dr David Spiegel, who conducted the study, was himself stunned by the findings, as was the medical community (Spiegel et al. 1989). Women with advanced breast cancer who went to weekly meetings with others survived twice as long as those with the same disease who faced it on their own. All the women received standard medical care, the only difference being that group members were able to unburden themselves with others who understood what they faced and were willing to listen to their fears, their pain and their anger. Often this was the only place where the women could be open about these emotions because other people in their lives dreaded talking about cancer and their imminent death. Women who did not participate in groups died on average in nineteen months, while those who attended the groups lived on average for thirty-seven additional months. This addition to their life expectancy was beyond the reach of any medication or other medical treatment. Had a new drug been responsible, pharmaceutical companies would have been battling to produce it. Such evidence suggests that a humane medical attitude that takes into consideration the patient's feelings is not just a luxury and optional extra but constitutes good medical practice.

AN EXAMPLE OF CARING FOR A PATIENT IN THE
GENERAL PRACTICE SETTING

Frank: The Patient's Physical Symptoms

Frank was fifty-eight years old when he presented to me one morning in June, complaining that there was blood in his urine. This strong, healthy man had rarely attended the surgery before. He was very frightened because the sight of blood in his urine made him think immediately of cancer. I was moved by his fear and wanted to reassure him. Even though cancer was a possibility and he needed to be investigated urgently, there are many causes of blood in the urine and many have a better prognosis. I explained all this to him and sent a specimen of his urine to the laboratory for examination. I wrote a referral letter for an urgent appointment to the urology department, and while waiting for the results of the test I gave him a course of antibiotics in case the blood in the urine was due to an infection. Three days later he came back in a panic and said that he could not wait for the appointment and wanted something done about his problem immediately. I responded to his distress by arranging for the specialist to see him urgently in Casualty later that day.

His Worst Fear is Realised

I did not hear anything about Frank until, two months later, a letter from the consultant urologist informed me that he had found a mass in his left kidney that he planned to remove in a month's time. His wife Irene, also a patient of ours, came to see me at the practice in a distressed state two days before his operation. She told me that she could not take in that Frank had cancer. Her father had died of cancer of the brain twenty years earlier and she was aware of the awful prognosis. She was worried that Frank might die on the operating table, and said that some husbands you want to get rid of but her husband was an angel and she did not want him to die. She asked me to sign her off work because she was too distressed to concentrate. I tried to comfort her and told her that cancer is not necessarily a death sentence, that modern treatments are very effective and that some cancers are curable. I invited her to come to see me regularly at the practice to talk about her fears. She came back a week after Frank's operation, greatly relieved that God had answered her prayers and he had come through. She remembered that after her mother's death she had developed Irritable Bowel Syndrome which had lasted for fifteen years; and after her father's death she had developed tingling in her tongue which lasted for four years. She was now afraid that if Frank died she herself would become ill. She had always relied on him for everything, for paying the bills and managing the finances. She could not imagine living without him.

The Assault on Hope

Three weeks after the operation Frank's son rang me at the surgery and asked me to visit his father at home because he had been feeling cold since the operation. He was abrupt and forceful, and when I asked him whether his father knew that he was requesting a visit on his behalf he exploded angrily that he could not discuss his worry with his father, and besides, his father was not the kind of person who would worry a doctor with his complaints and would I go and visit him immediately. I was annoyed with him for giving me orders but on reflection I could understand his aggression as being related to the shock of his father's illness. I rang Frank to confirm that he wanted to see me, and went to visit him after the evening surgery.

I found him looking fearful rather than ill. His wound was healing well but was still sore on examination. I could find no evidence of infection or other complication of his surgery and encouraged him to talk about his feelings. At once he burst into tears and talked about his frustration and rage that he could not do what he used to do. Every movement was painful and he was still not able to come to terms with the double shock of having cancer followed by a major operation. I acknowledged his feelings and read to him the consultant's letter confirming that he had removed the whole tumour and his hope that that would be the end of it. On my way out of the door he mentioned in passing that he had had some pain on his right shoulder since the operation for which the hospital doctors had given him painkillers. I reassured him by saying that he must have hurt his shoulder during the operation. For the doctors to remove his left kidney he must have been lying on his right side for some time. I invited him to come to the surgery with his wife regularly to talk about their fears and worries.

Two weeks later they both came to see me. Frank showed me his right collar bone which had become swollen. I examined him and felt dismayed. I said nothing to him but knew that the swelling could be nothing else but a secondary. I sent him for a chest X-ray immediately. The radiologist telephoned me the same day to confirm that the X-rays showed that the cancer had spread to his clavicle and lungs. I could not bear to tell Frank the bad news, so I arranged for him to see the urology registrar at the hospital in three days time. After their visit to the hospital I had a telephone call from Frank's son in the middle of my surgery furiously demanding to know why his father's secondaries had not been picked up earlier. He had been complaining of shoulder pain for several weeks and nobody had taken it seriously. The doctor who saw him at the hospital told him that he had secondaries, that there was nothing more they could do for him, and that he was going to die in a year! She had given him painkillers and sent him home. The son said that he would not let the matter rest there and demanded to find out why the doctors were so negligent.

I was taken aback by this aggressive onslaught, felt confused and did not know what to say. I felt guilty because I had not thought of secondaries when Frank complained to me of shoulder pain a few weeks before and had not taken any action. I tried to say something comforting and blurted out rather inappropriately that at least his father had had a few weeks of hope. That seemed to be the wrong thing to say. He was so beside himself with rage that he could not talk to me any more. ' I cannot believe what the man is saying', I heard him hissing as he passed the telephone receiver to his wife. I could hear him swearing in the background and I was frightened. When I put the receiver down I was seized by a strong fear that this man could seek me out and attack me physically or even kill me. I had heard of obstetricians who had been shot by the enraged husbands of women who had died in childbirth and immediately telephoned the consultant to discuss the family's anger and distress. He responded by offering to refer Frank to an oncologist/radiotherapist for further treatment.

I was afraid for my life for a week and tried to modulate my fear by reflecting on it. At the time, I thought of my fear of being killed as a result of the inability of the family to come to terms with the possibility of Frank's death, which aroused my own fear of dying.

It was not until a week later, when Frank, Irene and their son came to see me jointly, that I understood my fear of being killed as a response to the family's murderous rage. They were very angry with the hospital registrar who, in a cold and unempathic way, had told them that Frank had a year to live. Frank said that he had been given a death sentence, an execution order. He was not given any hope for any treatment. He felt that if he was a weaker man he would have been tempted to finish it all there and then.

Elizabeth Kübler Ross (1969) has written that all her patients were nourished by hope. They showed their greatest confidence in the doctors who allowed for this hope – realistic or not – and appreciated it when hope was offered, in spite of bad news. This does not mean that their doctors have to tell them a lie but merely that they share with them the hope that something unforeseen may happen, that they may have a remission, or that they might live longer than expected. It is a fact that we all know that we are going to die; what we do not know is the exact time and way of our death. Were we to know the exact time and circumstances of our death we might be too afraid, too discouraged, too paralysed to live a meaningful life. These thoughts helped me to understand my fear of being killed as an emotional response to the murderous rage caused by the assault on hope. Fortunately Frank recovered his own hope on starting radiotherapy which stopped the destruction of his clavicle. His experience with the hospital registrar made him say that he had to fight for his treatment.

As he had hinted at the intense mental suffering that he could not share with Irene, I invited him to come and see me on his own for a 'man to man' talk, as he put it. During this talk, I heard that he was trying hard to be strong for Irene's sake. He could not discuss his fears with her or cry in front of her.

Since the hospital registrar told him that he had a year to live, he had had a recurrent dream that he was swimming in a sea of oil. When he was knee-deep in it, a black cloud began to cover the sky from one end of the horizon to the other. 'The black cloud of despair', I commented. 'Yes', he said and burst into tears.

His Wife's Physical Symptoms

A month after he was told he was going to die Frank and Irene came to the surgery together. Irene said she was going to pieces. After forty years of marriage she had developed an allergy to her wedding ring! It had started burning her finger and she had to take it off. She showed me a ring of redness where her wedding ring had been. She had also been coughing all the time and could not sleep. I realised the symbolic significance of her symptoms but I decided not to make any interpretations. The combination of symptoms suggested the involvement of her immune system and I treated her with topical steroids for the contact dermatitis and inhaled steroids for the cough, as though she had asthma. Her symptoms diminished quickly and after a few weeks she was able to put the ring on her finger again.

This was the only time Irene went to pieces. She found the strength to nurse her husband and to maintain her feelings at tolerable levels of intensity by keeping her house immaculately tidy and clean.

Intolerable Emotions

However, black clouds were gathering on the horizon. Six weeks after their joint visit to the surgery, Frank complained of pain in his spine and a few days later his left arm fractured spontaneously as he was getting into his car. This was obviously the effect of another bone secondary and he was admitted to hospital where his arm was fixed with a plate and pins. A bone scan showed secondaries in his spine.

When I visited him at his home after his discharge a month later he was frightened and uncomfortable. His movements had become painful and getting in and out of bed with a broken arm was difficult. He needed his wife's help more and more. He was started on interferon injections, a new treatment for his type of cancer, which, although it gave him hope for a remission, made him suffer with debilitating influenza-like symptoms lasting two or three days after each injection. As he had two injections weekly he had very little time symptom-free. Thinking of the difficulties ahead I suggested that I contact the terminal care Macmillan team to provide extra support for his increasing symptoms and nursing needs. As soon as he heard the name he was convulsed with sobs. I reassured him that involving the Macmillan service does not mean that everything is lost, but obtaining extra help for his wife to look after him. As his physical display of fear was so severe I offered to visit him again for another 'man to man' talk in order to help him express his fears in words in the hope of containing them.

Even though Frank was so scared of the implications of involving the Macmillan service, I discussed his problem with the medical director of the local hospice where the Macmillan team is based and asked for an application form which would also put him on the waiting list for a bed at the hospice in case he needed it when the time came.Two days later I was asked to visit Frank because he was in great pain. I was dismayed; not again, I thought. Driving to his home I came to a T-junction. Instead of turning left towards his home I turned right towards the hospice which is in our locality. I was annoyed that I had not yet received the application form and my conscious thought was to go to the hospice in order to fill it in on the spot.

Suddenly I was struck by the absurdity of my actions. Even if I did fill the application form that day it would take several days before it was processed. I was simply wasting time. I was delaying the painful task of confrontation with therapeutic impotence, and postponing the painful tasks of giving more bad news, of tolerating his fear, his anxiety and his despair, as well as those of his wife. I wished I could admit him to the hospice immediately so that this painful task was taken away from me. Or perhaps I wanted to take refuge in the hospice myself.

It was then that I thought of Christ's words when he was praying in the garden of Gethsemane before his ordeal. 'My father, if it be possible let this cup pass from me; nevertheles, not as I will but as thou wilt.' When I became aware of my wish to avoid being confronted with all this pain I realised that my task was indeed limited. All I had to do was assess the clinical condition and decide whether he needed admission or not. I was able then to accept my limited suffering, turn my car round and drive to his home.

He was in bed. He could not stand up. Examining his right leg I found that any movement caused great pain in his hip and I wondered whether he had sustained another pathological fracture, or whether he was about to do so. Somehow the thought of him fracturing his femur as he was going downstairs was horrible. I told him that he needed to go into hospital to find out whether he had another secondary. He looked at me disheartened: 'How long have I got, doctor?', he asked me. I told him that I did not think he was dying now any more than when he had broken his clavicle or his arm. They would treat him with radiotherapy and the pain would go.

At the hospital his pain was controlled with a cordal block which diminished the strength of his legs so that he could not get up without help any more. I visited him a few days after his discharge a month later: he looked at me sadly. 'Look at the state of me', he said. He was unable to get out of bed or walk; he felt like an eighty-year-old pensioner. He was convulsed with sobs. I encouraged him to talk about his feelings: the rage at his diminishing powers, the humiliation of having his bottom wiped by his wife, his fear, his disappointment that he would not be able to enjoy the retirement for which he had been saving for a visit to his wife's relatives in New Zealand. He felt as helpless as a baby that his wife could not lift. I listened attentively. Finally, I touched him on the shoulder and said unconvincingly: 'Don't despair; there is hope.' I told him that just as the swelling of his clavicle disappeared after radiotherapy, so it was probable that the secondaries in his spine and arm would disappear as well. I arranged to visit him regularly every Monday and I left.

His Doctor's Physical Symptoms

For the following two days I felt unwell, having developed a headache and a sore throat. I reflected on my symptoms and I identified them as the physical accompaniments of my sadness and, more disturbingly, as a regressive trend set in motion by an identification with Frank's helplessness. Frank continued to deteriorate. The Macmillan service had become involved, much to my relief, and Frank had another admission to the hospital for correction of his anaemia and high blood calcium. Soon after his discharge I was called to visit him because his legs had become suddenly swollen, an indication that an abdominal mass was interfering with the return of the blood from his legs. The oncologist considered that neither radiotherapy nor chemotherapy could shrink the tumour in his abdomen and that further hospital treatment was not advisable. Frank had entered the terminal phase of his cancer and if nursing him at home became unmanageable he should be admitted to the hospice.

As already mentioned, I had arranged to visit Frank every Monday after my morning surgery. The next such occasion was a Bank Holiday. When I woke up, I started to make plans to take my daughter swimming without any thought of Frank. As I bent over the sink to wash my face I felt a severe pain in my lower back, and fell onto my knees. Every movement was excruciatingly painful. The only position that was comfortable was lying down. I was shocked by the sudden onset of pain and I burst into tears. I did not know whether I was crying with pain or out of frustration for my helplessness, or at carrying such a heavy clinical responsibility from which I could not escape even on a Bank Holiday. The burden seemed too much. I had forgotten to arrange an alternative day to visit Frank and I realised that he would expect me to visit that Monday as usual. I could have telephoned him to postpone the visit until the following day but I was not at all sure that I would be feeling any better. I could not bear the thought of letting him down and not visiting him when he expected. As the day went on, the pain improved and by midday I could sit up. As it was still too painful to drive, my wife offered to drive me to Frank's home at noon, the usual time for my visits.

He showed me his legs and burst into tears. He was afraid that he might not be able to walk again. Sometimes he felt he could lie in bed for another fifteen or twenty years, but sometimes he was not all sure that he would be there next week. He felt weaker and weaker every day. He talked about his uncertainty and fear. He avoided crying in front of his wife because it upset her so much. So he bottled it up and had to let go from time to time. He was grateful to his wife who was so good and devotedly did everything for him. She was 'perhaps too devoted', he said, sobbing. I was very moved and thought of my own devoted wife who was waiting patiently for me in the car outside Frank's house. I encouraged him to take every day as it came and enjoy the things that still gave him pleasure, such as the sweets for which he had developed a craving. On my way out I had a brief talk with Irene, who did not know where she found the strength to cope. She wondered why Frank was punished in this way. 'He never did anything wrong. There are some bad people that no harm ever comes to ... .' I told her that cancer respects nobody. Innocent children can suffer from it; good men and bad men alike. It is the luck of the draw. She told me how helpless she felt witnessing Frank's prolonged agony. Some people die instantly with a heart attack. 'And yet', I pointed out, 'this long illness has brought you closer. You are able to show him how much you love him. Your devotion and care are his greatest comfort and you must not underestimate how important you have been. You cannot cure his cancer, medicine cannot cure his cancer, we cannot put the clock back; but you are always there when he needs you and this is the greatest help you can give him.' We were both in tears by then.

Don't Say Goodbye

I was off work for one week with my back pain and during that week the Macmillan team admitted Frank to the hospice because it had become impossible for Irene to lift him without causing him excruciating pain. She telephoned me during my emergency Saturday morning surgery to tell me what had happened. I went to visit him at the hospice after morning surgery. His deterioration was visible. He had lost a lot of weight, his speech was slurred and he was too exhausted to lift his arms; he had to be fed. Irene was trying to persuade the doctors to investigate his calcium levels because last time he had felt very ill and his hypercalcaemia had been treated, he had felt a lot better. She could still not accept that Frank might die. She could not imagine life without him. It was all so unfair. But I was reassured to hear that she was thinking of visiting her sister in New Zealand when it was all over.

I visited Frank again the next Monday. He was very pleased to see me. He said that I was a doctor in a million for always coming to see him. Irene kept thanking me for being so good to Frank. I had another talk with her, praising her for her attentive care and expressing my admiration for her devotion. I stressed again that she could not take the cancer away but her devoted attention was the greatest help and comfort she could give him.

A week later Frank had deteriorated dramatically. He could not swallow any more and his painkillers were being given subcutaneously with a drive pump. They all thought he was going to die over the weekend but miraculously he pulled through. When I next saw him it was obvious that he had only hours to live. I wanted to cry. 'Goodbye', I blurted out. He sobbed and squeezed my hand. 'No ... Don't say good bye.' 'OK', I replied. 'I will not say goodbye ... See you on Monday.' 'Yes, yes, see you on Monday', he echoed. I squeezed his hand. Irene was in tears. It was time to go. I expressed again my admiration for her courage, her stamina and the support she was giving him and asked her to let me know when Frank died. He died the following Friday. His illness had lasted eleven months from the onset of his first symptoms to his death. The estimate of one year by the urology registrar had been correct, but her attitude had been so insensitive. I also wondered what I had done to earn Frank's praise and gratitude. After all, compared to the hospital doctors I was as helpless and impotent in the fight against cancer as Irene.

Again, Elizabeth Kübler Ross's words come to mind. 'If the doctor sits and listens and repeats his visits, the patient will soon develop a feeling of confidence that here is a person who cares who is available and sticks around.' This function of the doctor has a holding quality. It helps to contain the anxiety, fear and despair of the patient and his family, so that they do not feel abandoned when they are so vulnerable. The doctor who can tolerate his own fear of death and reflect on the emotions aroused by the dying patient is in a position to communicate with the patient at a deep level, relieving his sense of isolation.

DO PHYSICAL SYMPTOMS HAVE MEANING?

The relatives and carers of a patient with severe physical disease are exposed not only to the fear and despair of the patient but also to their own painful emotional responses as they resonate with his feelings. When these feelings become very painful and difficult to tolerate, it is not unusual for the person to develop somatic symptoms that need treatment in their own right. For example, both Irene and I developed distressing physical symptoms at different times during Frank's illness, when our feelings became too intense and difficult to tolerate. She developed contact dermatitis to her wedding ring and a persistent cough, and I developed severe back pain that lasted for a few days.

The word somatisation has been coined to describe the behaviour of patients who ignore the emotional setting within which the somatic sensations arise, cannot make sense of their physical symptoms and keep consulting the doctor about their possible medical significance.

Do these symptoms have a meaning?

This is a controversial question that, as Graeme Taylor has emphasised in *Disorders of Affect Regulation* (Taylor et al. 1997), is as old as psychosomatic medicine itself.

The early psychosomatic doctors had a tendency to understand a physical disorder as an expression of a deep-seated neurosis and regarded somatisation as equivalent to the concept of conversion introduced by Breuer and Freud to explain the motor and sensory symptoms of hysteria (Breuer and Freud 1893). According to this view, physical symptoms have primary symbolic meaning comparable to the symptoms of conversion hysteria, for they represent a defence mechanism keeping conflicts over drive-related wishes and associated dysphoric affects unconscious, yet at the same time permitting their partial expression and gratification through bodily symptoms.

Somatisation and hypochondriasis provided ways of deflecting sexual, aggressive or oral drives as well as being defences against guilt or low self-esteem. Vaillant emphasised the transformation of aggressive and hostile impulses into hypochondriacal complaints; these impulses were presumed to stem from past disappointments, but achieved partial expression through the patient's complaining and reproaching other people for their suffering (Vaillant 1993). Other psychoanalytic theorists have conceptualised somatic symptoms and hypochondriacal complaints as an expression of pregenital wishes for caring, nurturance, attention, sympathy and physical contact. Somatic symptoms have also been thought of as a defence against awareness of certain personality deficiencies and as serving the need for atonement and punishment for past wrongdoings and a sense of inner badness. In other words, like psychoneurotic symptoms, functional somatic symptoms were considered to have symbolic meaning as well as defensive functions and to provide both primary and secondary gains.

Most psychosomatic doctors merely adopted the prevailing psychoanalytic view that emotions are drive derivatives and failed to consider that some patients might manifest arrests in affect development and associated deficits in affect regulation.

An alternative psychosomatic model that emphasised a role for affects in the onset of disease was introduced by Engel and Schmale (1967). Through studying patients with a wide variety of diseases and by shifting their focus of enquiry from intrapsychic conflicts to the life setting in which people become ill, these authors discovered that the onset or exacerbation of disease is associated frequently with the affects of helplessness and hopelessness evoked by a recent separation or loss of an important relationship.

They postulated that there is a heightened susceptibility to disease in individuals who are unable to grieve, or otherwise cope with separations and other object losses. Such individuals develop the specific depressive affects of helplessness and hopelessness, attitudes of giving up and having given up and a conservation/withdrawal physiological response. They called this intervening psychobiological state the giving up/given up complex. They postulated that once the complex develops, it initiates autonomic, endocrinologic and immunologic changes that may lead to the emergence of disease if the necessary constitutional and environmental factors are also present.

In exploring why some disease-prone individuals adapt poorly to separations and other object losses, Engel identified defects in 'ego function' which appeared to stem from developmental arrests and were compensated for by excessive dependency on a symbiotic relationship. The disruption of such a relationship exposed the defects in the personality, including an inability to modulate the negative affects evoked by the loss.

Recent developments in neuropsychobiology and the science of emotions have favoured the view that functional somatic symptoms are the consequence of defective emotional processing rather than being the symbolic expression of a drive-related conflict.

However, when the subject is faced with a somatic symptom of such obvious symbolic meaning as Irene's allergic reaction to her wedding ring, we realise that the two psychosomatic models are not mutually exclusive but rather that the disregulation model is overarching.

Of course, it is one thing for the therapist to detect a symbolic meaning in a psychosomatic symptom and another for the patient to discover the meaning for herself. The meaning of psychosomatic symptoms relates to the strong feelings aroused by life events, which may not be recognised as such by the subject because they are too primitive to be expressed in words, or too painful or shameful, or because they create feelings of guilt. The physiological arousal and heightened autonomic activity associated with strong emotions can not only be experienced as functional symptoms, but may produce conditions conducive to the development of somatic disease if this activity is prolonged and not adequately regulated. Those who are aware that their somatic symptoms are the direct consequence of the way they feel find it much easier to regulate and tolerate their emotions.

We may infer Irene's feelings from her phrase that her husband was an angel and she did not want him to die. Bettelheim (Bettelheim and Rosenfeld 1993), has taught that when a person refers to a relative as an angel, it sounds as if she is telling us how good he is. But in a subtle way she is expressing her ambivalence about the real him, or their relationship, which cannot be all that good. Angels live in heaven and to become an angel one has to die first. Irene had to come to terms with a very complex set of emotions; not only with the sorrow aroused by the imminent loss of her husband and the possible unfinished business from the death of her own parents that it reactivated, but also with the anger and fear evoked by her imminent abandonment by the person she depended on and who was becoming progressively more dependent on her. She also had to deal with the helplessness that his progressive deterioration and suffering aroused in her and possibly her guilt for wishing an early end to this.

Although it is tempting to speculate that the allergy to the wedding ring symbolised the suffering in her marriage or even the rejection of that suffering, all I can say with any confidence is that the contact dermatitis occurred within a context of helplessness, not only with regard to Frank's inexorable physical deterioration but also with regard to the overwhelming and unwanted negative emotions it aroused.

My therapeutic aim, therefore, was to counter Irene's helplessness by acknowledging and encouraging the power of her capacity to tolerate her emotions and to stand by her dying husband.

I believe that developing an interest in the way emotions influence the body makes us more tolerant of our feelings and the feelings of our patients.

3   HOW DO EMOTIONS INFLUENCE THE BODY?

Griefs, at the moment when they change into ideas, lose some of their power to injure the heart.

Marcel Proust, *À la recherche du temps perdu.*

THREE PSYCHOSOMATIC MODELS

Although the idea that emotions can influence our body and our health has been prominent among philosophers since antiquity, it was the development of psychoanalysis at the beginning of the twentieth century that gave the impetus for a systematic study of the relationship between mind and body.

The early psychoanalysts began to study the personality and psychological traits that were assumed to be responsible for the emotional states contributing to the development of disease. Their work led to the emergence of psychosomatic medicine as an organised movement and to the founding of the various psychosomatic societies.

Psychosomatic medicine is an evolving discipline but its subject remains controversial. There is disagreement even about whether one should use a hyphen between the words psycho and somatic.

Donald Winnicott, one of the most original and innovative English psychoanalysts, begins his classic paper: 'Psycho-somatic illness in its positive and negative aspects' by asserting that the 'word psycho-somatic is needed because no simple word exists which is appropriate to describe certain clinical states. The hyphen both joins and separates the two aspects of medical practice which are constantly under review in any discussion of this theme and the word accurately describes something that is inherent in this work' (Winnicott 1964).

Anthony Storr, a Jungian psychoanalyst and a lifelong asthmatic, introducing Dr Donald Lane's book *Asthma: The Facts*, confesses that 'many of us have given up using the term psychosomatic in the belief that it is a cloak for ignorance rather than a description of any value' (Lane and Storr 1981).

The initial surprise at such discrepant views between senior psychoanalysts becomes intelligible only when we realise that Anthony Storr's criticism is levelled at the first psychosomatic model only and not at the general idea that emotions or stress can influence the body. To appreciate this point we have to take a historical perspective of the changing meaning of the term 'psychosomatic' over the years, as our knowledge of biology and psychology is expanding.

With the great medical scientific discoveries of the nineteenth and twentieth centuries many doctors became entirely preoccupied with physical and technical considerations in treating disease. The concept of psychosomatic medicine was originally used to counteract this tendency and to remind them to treat not only the disease, but also the person by paying equal attention to the psychological, social and biological aspects of illness and their interaction. However, interest in psychosomatic medicine gradually declined until Freud described the psychological mechanism responsible for the development of physical symptoms in conversion hysteria, after which the interest in psychosomatic medicine revived.

The First Model

Psychosomatic medicine flourished in the 1940s and 1950s. The understanding of psychosomatic disorders was based on the psychoanalytic concept of unconscious psychic conflict, derived from the treatment of psychoneurotic patients.

Franz Alexander, a Chicago psychoanalyst, used the term 'psychosomatic illness' for a small group of seven diseases associated with demonstrable structural changes in body organs, in which psychological factors were thought to play an important aetiological role. These were peptic ulcer, ulcerative colitis, bronchial asthma, thyrotoxicosis, rheumatoid arthritis, essential hypertension and eczema (Alexander 1950).

Alexander's work gave rise to the *intrapsychic conflict model*. He postulated a mobilisation of powerful emotions by environmental events interacting with a predisposition based on past history and genetic factors. The emotions so aroused were blocked from expression by equally powerful inhibitory forces similarly derived. So he believed, for example, that asthma took origin from a particular conflict, starting in childhood, between deep dependence upon the mother and fear of becoming estranged from her by somehow offending her by sexual desire or a drive for independence. Blocked urges to cry might contribute to an asthmatic attack which helps re-establish the threatened bond to the mother (Alexander and French 1946).

The Second Model

The second model was called the *pregenital symbolism model* by Fenichel and was originally described by Groddeck (1977) and Deutsch (1945). It emphasises the symbolic meaning conveyed by the symptoms. For example, Peter Knapp, a president of the American Psychosomatic Society, hypothesised that the 'asthmatic state' consists of conflicting fantasies, regressively mobilised, in which destructive urges and emotions are inhibited by guilt and fear, while primitive urges to take in, retain and eliminate through the respiratory apparatus, are accentuated (Knapp 1989).

Despite the elegance of the above models, researchers soon became disillusioned with them because they were derived from the study of a very small number of patients and their therapeutic effectiveness was very limited.

The Third Model

Over the past twenty years, however, a number of researchers and theorists have attempted to integrate the recent exciting discoveries in the biological sciences with advances in our understanding of emotional development, and have elaborated the *disregulation model* which conceptualises many medical illnesses and diseases as disorders of psychobiological regulation. The essence of the disregulation model is its conception of human beings as self-regulating cybernetic systems. Each person is made up of a hierarchy of reciprocally regulating subsystems that interface via the brain with the larger social system. There is ample evidence that these subsystems regulate each other's activities as well as their own. Recent research, for instance, has shown that not only can the neuroendocrine system regulate immune functions but also that the immune system can regulate neuroendocrine functions (Watkins 1997). Graeme Taylor has written extensively about this paradigm shift in our understanding of psychosomatic relationships (Taylor 1987, Taylor et al. 1997).

In the disregulation model of psychosomatic medicine, the separation between mind and body falls away when the organism is seen as a dynamic communication system of information processing and exchange which regulates its own behaviour and that of its components in response to an internal signalling system. Emotional responding, which in humans communicates simultaneously in chemical, body and verbal language, is such a signalling system.

According to Herbert Weiner, professor of psychiatry and biobehavioural sciences at the school of medicine and brain research institute at the University of California, the advantage of viewing the organism in this way is that a common language may describe the part and whole functions of the organism. In this framework, both verbal language and body language are communication signals and they perform analogous functions to the chemical language of hormones and neurotransmitters (Weiner 1989).

At this point it is important to emphasise that the three psychosomatic models are not mutually exclusive but rather that the third is overarching both, as the example in the first chapter has illustrated.

THE THREE LANGUAGES OF EMOTIONS

The subjective experience of relief, when the intensity of an affect subsides, has given rise to the discharge metaphor of emotion. As Henry Krystal (1988) has pointed out, however, the metaphors of discharge we use when we refer to emotions have made our understanding of emotions difficult. The phrase 'Help the patient to express his emotions' plays into the desire of many people to rid themselves of undesirable parts, to vent their emotions and get rid of them. Indeed, Freud's original view of emotions was that they represented physiological discharge phenomena which could become attached to ideas. According to his early view, affects were the conscious manifestations of instincts and represented a quantitative accumulation of discharge. His entire original theory of anxiety described a model of converting libido into affect for the purpose of discharge. However, Michael Basch, in his paper 'The re-examination of the concept of affect', has argued that Freud towards the end of his life broke down the barrier between affect and cognition by recognising anxiety as being always a signal of impending danger rather than an indicator of discharge (Basch 1976). This view is in agreement with the modern way of understanding emotions which views them as communication signals which are valuable parts of ourselves and are essential for survival.

Although the study of emotion is an area of science which is full of controversy, most researchers agree that emotions are complex and multi-faceted phenomena. There is a strong consensus among researchers that emotions are characterised by three responses which carry their whole informational and signal contents.

The Chemical Language

The chemical language response is a neuroendocrine response (autonomic nervous system and neuroendocrine activation) which uses the chemical language of hormones and neurotransmitters to communicate with other parts of the organism. This includes the physiological manifestations of emotions such as sweating, increase in heart rate, changes in breathing pattern, changes in gut activity, shedding of tears, and so on.

One of William James's lasting contributions to the science of emotion is that emotions do create signals in the body which return to the brain as a somatic feedback, contribute to the development of emotional awareness and give each emotion its unique quality. When we become aware of the visceral sensations of emotional arousal we use such expressions as 'butterflies' in our stomach, feeling 'gutted', having a 'gut-wrenching' feeling, having a 'sinking' feeling, feeling 'drained', and so on.

Psychoneuroimmunologists have discovered recently that the hormones corticotrophin releasing factor, cortisol and a number of cytokines are essential for the regulation of both the stress and the immune response. In other words, at least the emotions of fear and anger and the immune system share the same chemical language (Sternberg and Gold 1997).

The Body Language

The body language response is a behavioural response that relates to the impulse to express an emotion in action and is communicated through body language. This includes motor-expressive behaviours such as facial expressions, gestures, body posture and the emotional inflection of the voice. The inflection is an instance of prosody, the musical, tonal accompaniments to the speech sounds that constitute the words.

It is possible for the emotional message contained in the prosody of the speech to contradict the verbal message. For instance, one can enquire about somebody's health in a prosody that unmistakably registers indifference or even hostility.

The neurophysiological and behavioural responses usually operate outside awareness and are part of our emotional unconscious.

The Verbal Language

The verbal language response is a cognitive response which is communicated through verbal language and refers to the thoughts and fantasies we have when we are in the grip of an emotion, as well as the meaning and the story behind that emotion. For instance, the thought that we may have been wronged by another person may accompany the emotion of anger. Also, both anxiety and fear signal the perception of impending danger. Their meaning is: 'Something bad is about to happen.' But the story behind them is different. Fear refers to the possibility of external danger in actuality, whereas anxiety refers to some danger deriving from within oneself. The story behind distress or sadness may contain a nucleus of a loss that is frequently buried by various self-blaming and complaining responses, beneath which may be an ambivalent relationship to the person who has been lost. Unconscious anger is one of the determinants of unfinished, unresolved mourning.

It is obvious from the above discussion that emotions are simultaneously both somatic and psychological and therefore bridge the mind–body divide. Their study is vital in understanding mind–body links.

THE FOUR THEORETICAL TRADITIONS IN EMOTION RESEARCH

There are four theoretical traditions in emotion research, according to which response is considered primary. Randolph Cornelius, in his concise book *The Science of Emotion*, has given a superb summary of all of them (Cornelius 1996).

The Darwinian tradition is based on Darwin's observation that the facial and bodily display of certain emotions is similar in human babies, adults, across cultures and in certain apes. He proposed that some discrete emotions manifest themselves through distinct patterns of facial expressions and body language which occur in a reflex-like manner and result from the direct action of the central nervous system. He understood these to be communication signals important for social adaptation and survival.

The Jamesian tradition is inspired by James's insistence that the experience of emotion is primarily the experience of bodily changes.

The cognitive tradition emphasises the role of thought in the genesis of emotion and focuses on the way emotions follow from the manner in which individuals appraise events in the environment (the process of judging the personal significance of an event for good or ill).

Finally, the social constructivist tradition emphasises that emotions are cultural constructions that serve particular social and individual ends and can only be understood by attending to a social level of analysis.

Of all the above traditions, however, the Darwinian and Jamesian traditions, which view emotions as primarily biological phenomena, are particularly important for understanding mind–body links (Pally 1998).

A VOCABULARY FOR THINKING AND TALKING ABOUT EMOTIONS

A Clinical Example: Joyce

Joyce was fifteen years old when her mother brought her to see me because she was suffering from low abdominal pain.

She had a mature expression, looked serious and spoke with a faint ironic smile. I felt attracted to her personality. The pain had started three days previously as an ache and gradually got sharper. The pain hurt in the middle of her tummy and when she drank or ate anything she felt sick. The pain was waxing and waning in character and when it got bad she felt hot and developed a headache.

This was the third episode of abdominal pain. When she had had the first one four months previously, it was so bad that she was admitted to hospital where, after five days of intensive investigations, no abnormality was found. She was admitted to another hospital following the second episode where a doctor told her that there was nothing wrong with her and that she was making things up. She was very upset by this. After a physical examination I was able to explain to mother and daughter that the pains suggested the diagnosis of Irritable Bowel Syndrome and invited them to come again with a longer appointment in order to go into the history in some more detail.

A week later Joyce came back on her own, and as I was taking her family history I found out that her father had died of AIDS two years previously and that she had nursed him during the last two months of his life.

I was astonished and moved. She told me that she was at his home from 8 a.m. to 10 p.m. during the weekends and used to visit him after school during the weekdays. She was told of his diagnosis one year before he died. She looked it up and read a lot about it. She watched him gradually getting thinner and thinner, but she saw him only as her dad.

I asked her how his death affected her and she told me, in a calm, matter of fact voice, that she had blanked out all the memories around his funeral and for several days after it. She did not remember what she did or how she reacted. Her mother told her that she had not cried enough.

I wondered how big a gap her father had left in her life as she had been visiting him every day for two months. She agreed that he was always there for her. She could tell him anything. She used to ring him every day, too. When he died she went to ring him and he was not there.

As she was talking of her father, her eyes became wet and a tear started rolling down her left cheek. She wiped it off mechanically, as if she were chasing off an annoying fly.

Then she told me that her father was gay and he found out that he was HIV positive two months after her parents separated when she was eighteen months old. When I asked how she felt about this she told me that for her he was her dad and she loved him.

Another tear started rolling down her left cheek and this time I pointed it out to her. She was surprised and did not believe me. But she touched her face and realised that indeed it was a tear. I told her that her eyes were crying as she was talking about her father and wondered whether she felt sad. 'No', she said. 'I do not.'

This intervention made it possible to suggest to her later that her abdominal pain was as real as her tears, the physical manifestation of an emotion that she could not feel.

Many people who hear the statement that tears are one of the most frequent psychosomatic symptoms become surprised, because they had not thought about tears in this way before. Although weeping is relatively easy to identify as one of the components of the crying response that is part of the affect of sadness, some of our patients are not aware of feeling sad when they weep. When this is the case, they may not be able to make sense of the state of their eyes and they may present to the doctor complaining of watering eyes or sore eyes. In general practice, we often meet patients who are in the grip of an affect without being aware that they are experiencing a feeling.

AFFECTS, EMOTIONS, FEELINGS, MOODS

In everyday language we use the terms 'affects', 'emotions', 'feelings' and 'moods' interchangeably. The result is confusion about the specific meaning of each word. Although we need an exact language for an exact science of emotions, there is no consensus at the moment about the definition of each of these terms.

Silvan Tomkins, professor at the department of Social Systems Sciences at the University of Pennsylvania, in a series of books called *Affect, Imagery and Consciousness*, has proposed such a working definition which is not yet accepted by all researchers in the field of affect research (Tomkins 1962, 1963, 1991, 1992).

According to Tomkins, the term *Affect* describes the strictly biological portion of emotion. To say that an affect has been activated is to say that some definable stimulus has triggered a mechanism which then releases a known pattern of biological events.

Each affect unfolds according to its own precisely written programme. Each lasts a strictly determined period of time ranging from a few hundredths of a second to a couple of seconds. These patterns are genetically transmitted, are present from birth, and there is evidence that they first appeared in life forms as primitive as the reptile. In humans their circuitry is stored in the primitive portion of the brain which Paul MacLean has called 'the reptile brain' (MacLean 1949).

An adult in the grip of an affect may get ready for action. He may clench his jaw and his fists and prepare to fight and shout when he is angry, he may feel cold and his muscles may become stiff when he is frightened, or he may avoid eye contact when he is embarrassed. The outward displays of emotion are accompanied by alterations in internal biological function. For instance, the heart beats faster during the moment of fear or anger; the face blushes during embarrassment.

In order for these large-scale events to occur a host of tiny events must take place at the microscopic and submicroscopic level. Electrochemical messages must travel along pathways within the central nervous system. The subcortical centres of the primitive brain organise these chemical signals into messages which dispose the organism toward adaptive actions. Affect, then, is another form of subcortically guided adaptation. Once it is identified as an adaptive behaviour, a form of communication mediated by the autonomic nervous system and relying primarily on chemical transmission of messages, a form of communication more general and rapid in its effects than is the transmission of signals in the associational cortex, it ceases to be a mysterious event and takes its place among the physiological processes and their psychological manifestations. Just being in the grip of an affect, however, does not mean that the person is aware of experiencing it and is able to name it and use it as information to himself.

The word *feeling* indicates that the person has become *aware* of an affect.

An animal may look startled when exposed to a loud noise, but only to the extent that a life form has the advanced brain mechanism needed to produce the degree of consciousness we call awareness will it be able to recognise that it has been gripped by an affect. Feeling implies the presence of higher order mechanisms or components that allow knowledge and understanding.

The infant's inborn automatic behaviour patterns with which it responds to stimulation have always been called affective because they provide the substrate for the eventual development of emotional experience which is an outgrowth of the later acquired symbolic function. Once conceptualisation becomes possible for human beings after the age of two and with the development of the capacity to describe concepts discursively through speech, translation of various behavioural patterns into emotional experiences begins. The capacity for conceptualising, describing and naming their feelings is still quite incomplete even in older children, though they show the full range of appropriate affective reaction.

Adults can also react affectively without necessarily experiencing a feeling. That is, they remain unaware of the significance of their reactions. For example, it is not uncommon for an observer to recognise that another person is responding angrily to a particular situation by observing the tone of voice, tightened jaw muscles, flushed face and narrowing of the eyes, while the subject of these observations may honestly be able to deny that he is conscious of the corresponding emotion. The affective reaction is clearly manifested and signalled, but the feeling, the reflective judgement made on the affective experience, is not present. The term *feeling* then refers to the awareness of the meaning of an affect for the self and is evidence of neocortical activity of a highly sophisticated form. Antonio Damasio, in *The Feeling of What Happens*, gives a comprehensive account of the neural mechanisms that make it possible for an affect to become a feeling (Damasio 1999).

The move from affect to feeling involves a leap from biology to psychology.

An *emotion* is the complex combination of an affect with the memories and affects they also trigger. So we can say that affect is biology, feeling is psychology and emotion is biography.

Donald Nathanson, professor of psychiatry and human behaviour at Jefferson Medical College and director of the Silvan Tomkins Institute, who has summarised the work of Tomkins in his book *Shame and Pride. Affect, Sex and the Birth of the Self*, emphasises that before the work of Tomkins most people neglected the biology of affect in favour of the historical path along which the affect had travelled. He claims that we have spent too much time studying biography and far too little on the biology that makes it possible (Nathanson 1992).

An affect lasts a few seconds; a feeling only long enough for us to make the flash of recognition; an emotion lasts as long as we keep finding memories that continue to trigger that affect.

Mood is a persistent emotional state in which we can remain stuck for hours or days. It can happen when our memories bring to our attention an unsolved problem from the past, such as the emotions about a relationship we never managed to resolve. If the combination of memories and feelings brings to our attention some part of our emotional life which we had hoped to ignore, and the weight of current sadness in combination with sadness past becomes more than can be dissipated, the emotion gives way to mood.

THE AFFECT SYSTEM

The study of the human body is made easier when it is subdivided into the various systems that constitute it. Even though the presence of most anatomical organs of the body was known from antiquity, it was only relatively recently that their integration into functional systems was made possible.

For example, in 1628 William Harvey's seminal anatomical essay on the 'motion of the heart and blood in animals' described his discovery of the cardiovascular system.

In 1893 Elie Metchnicoff recognised that certain specialised cells mediate defence against microbial infections, so fathering the whole concept of the immune system that guards the boundaries of what is us from what is alien to our cells.

Silvan Tomkins, who followed the Darwinian tradition, started in 1950 to describe the affect system. It is his work that I have found most useful in understanding the centrality of emotions for the meaning of some physical symptoms of my patients.

His theory began to develop with a burst of insight while observing his newborn son starting to cry. He realised then that crying is a complex series of behaviours. The eyes pour tears; the larynx makes a sound; the face and the eyes become red; the mouth takes a peculiar shape, the omega of melancholy. Tomkins realised that it was unlikely that his son had started to cry following a cognitive assessment of the world he was born into as a vale of tears. Most likely there was a script for crying, a programme that could be set off by some button. If the right button is pushed both in the adult and the child, then the crying response will be elicited. The cry is an organised behaviour with a precise form. Whatever allows an infant to cry must trigger something that allows the organised behaviour to start and then to unfold in its own particular way until it comes to an end.

The Components of the Affect System

The affect system, according to Tomkins, consists of four components: affects, receptors, effectors and mediators, and the scripts that are known as innate affects.

Affects

Affects are Urgent

Before Tomkins, it was considered that affect, behaviour and cognition represented three different functions of the human brain. Tomkins's work demonstrated that these distinctions are arbitrary and incorrect.

Affect causes behaviours throughout the body. Not only does affect influence and often control the thinking made possible by the most advanced structures of the new brain (the neocortex) but it is itself a form of thinking. It is the action thinking of the old brain. According to Tomkins, affects are triggered by meaning-free increases or decreases in the activity of the brain, or neural firing as he prefers to call it. For instance, an optimal increase in brain activity triggers the affect programme of interest, that causes an amplification of this optimal state of brain function. The triggering of affect takes what might be interesting and now makes it very interesting. This affect programme makes things happen all over the body, the effect of which is to add urgency to the increase in brain activity.

Affects are Abstract

Nothing about sobbing tells us anything about the steady state stimulus that triggered it. Sobbing itself has nothing to do with hunger or cold or loneliness. Only the fact that we grow up with an increasing experience of sobbing lets us form some ideas about its meaning.

Affects are Analogues

Each affect is analogic; it resembles what triggered it. Affects make bad things worse and good things better. Terror and rage were designed to amplify toxic states and make them worse, goading the individual to heroic emergency antitoxic responses. Affects that respond to intense constant levels of neural firing will themselves feel like an intense and constant but highly amplified level of activity.

The Stimulus Profile

Tomkins's basic idea is that the function of affect is to amplify the highly specific stimulus that set it in motion. A stimulus that involves an increase in the brain's activity will trigger an affect that increases brain activity. A stimulus that involves a decrease in brain activity will trigger an affect that further decreases this activity. The profile of stimulation is important. The affect that Tomkins called Surprise-Startle, for instance, is triggered by a hand clap or a pistol shot. A brief event is followed by a very brief affect. When the stimulus is constant and causes higher than optimal brain activity, the affect Distress-Anguish is triggered, the crying response, which is a constant density experience. If the stimulus causes an optimal increase in the intensity of brain activity the affect of interest will be triggered. When the stimulus increases in intensity at a rate that is less than is needed to produce surprise but greater than the optimal level capable of triggering interest, the innate affect of fear is activated. When the intensity of the stimulus is very high and remains high, it triggers Anger-Rage, as happens when we are exposed to very loud and intrusive noise.

Receptors

Each time an affect is triggered it creates information. The affect programme for fear does something to the hairs that changes them from their quiescent state to an erect state. Their follicles just a moment ago the site of action of an affect programme, now act as a sensory device transmitting to the brain the information that the organism is frightened. The affect system has receptors all over the body. The term 'receptors' may be used in this special sense to describe the places in the body where an affect can become a feeling.

In distress we cry, in fear our hair stands on end. Affect can alter patterns of secretion and movement in the gut. In fear some individuals are cotton-mouthed, others have diarrhoea or nausea. Pre-existing mechanisms may be triggered during the affect. The mechanisms of sweating, breathing and gut function can be taken over temporarily by affect.

Crying is more than weeping. Sobbing also involves the vocal expression of distress. The voice is a major instrument of the affect system. The adult can use affect-based expression to produce the emotional tonality that adds delicate shades of meaning to words. Every system of the body can become the target of affect and become involved in the experience of affect. The influence of affects on the cardiovascular, respiratory, gastrointestinal, endocrine and musculoskeletal system is well documented. The influence of affects on the immune system has only recently begun to be explored.

But by far the most important site of action for affect display is the face. The facial expression of affect involves voluntary muscles momentarily taken over by an involuntary mechanism. At the beginning of life, the infant becomes used to feeling these muscles captured by the affect programmes and sooner or later begins to play with these muscles of expression. Simulated affect expressions are themselves a real stimulus of affect. If mere simulated affect can produce real affect, then we must look more carefully at what is going on between caregiver and infant. Affect is extremely contagious.

Our current attitude to normal parenting requires that mothers remain available to the contagious quality of their babies' affect. The mother is unavoidably swept into her baby's affect, or she purposefully imitates the baby's facial expression. Instantly she begins to experience the same affect as the child. Suddenly they are in communication. By the simple process of imitation or the acceptance of contagion, the caregiver has entered the internal system of the baby. This is the beginning of empathy. During empathy we try each other's affect display which triggers a weak experience of innate affect, following which we bring to this affect our lifetime of remembered emotional experience in an attempt to appreciate the world of the other person. Affect provides the infant with a powerful link to the outside world.

Effectors and Mediators

The anatomical structures that carry the affective messages are the effectors. The stimulating chemicals are the mediators of affect. The brain is also an endocrine organ, a hormone factory of noradrenaline, serotonin and several other hormones and peptides. Compounds taken into the body for other reasons can become mediators of affect. For instance, methyldopa, prescribed for the treatment of hypertension, can cause depression, and the drug pseudoephedrine, that we prescribe for the control of symptoms of the common cold, can cause anxiety.

The structural effectors and the chemical mediators will carry messages to specific sites of action where receptors allow recognition of the patterns of affect activity.

The Innate Affects

Tomkins, following the Darwinian tradition, identified a small number of discrete innate affects by studying facial expressions. In addition he proposed that feedback from the muscles of the face was a major factor in differentiating between these affects. These innate affects are the final portion of the affect system and have to be thought of as a group of internal scripts, a group of hard wired pre-programmed, genetically transmitted mechanisms that exist in each one of us and are responsible for the earliest form of emotional life. These innate affects combine to form complex emotions and every known emotion and emotion laden situation can be explained on the basis of the nine innate affects described by Tomkins.

Positive Affects
Interest-Excitement
Enjoyment-Joy

Neutral Affect
Surprise-Startle

Negative Affects
Distress-Anguish
Shame-Humiliation
Fear-Terror
Anger-Rage
Disgust-Revulsion
Dissmell-Shunning

The idea that affect is experienced in degrees of intensity is so important to that of innate affect that Tomkins gave all of them paired names to indicate the range over which each might be experienced.

Affect System or Affect Systems?

This way of identifying emotions is contested at the moment by a number of neuroscientists, including Le Doux, who studies the foundation of memory and emotion at the centre of neural science at New York University. In his recent book *The Emotional Brain* (1998), Le Doux argues that attempts to find a single unified system of emotion have not been successful. Using the label emotional behaviour should not lead to the assumption that all labelled functions are mediated by one system in the brain. He believes that different emotions are mediated by different brain systems or networks and changes in a particular network do not necessarily affect the others directly. Rather than talking about basic emotions he prefers to talk about basic functions necessary for survival. Emotions are such functions, but since different emotions are involved in different survival functions each may well involve different brain systems. Seeing and hearing are both sensory functions but each has its own neural machinery. He believes that listing special adaptive behaviours crucial for survival would be a better way of producing an inventory of basic emotions than the more standard ways such as facial expressions, body responses and introspection. For example, at the first international neuro-psychoanalysis conference that took place in London in July 2000, Douglas Watt, a neuroscientist, pointed out that at present neuroscience supports three such neural systems which are highly complex and are intrinsically related. These are an organism defence system centred on fear and rage; a system that supports attachment behaviour and is responsible for the affects of sadness, guilt, shame and joy, and a system that supports exploratory behaviour and the affects of interest and curiosity and can be considered nature's way of saying 'Don't just sit there, do something.' There is no doubt that with the recent exponential development of neuroscience a consensus will have to be reached soon about the definition and classification of affects so that researchers of emotion from different fields can communicate in a common language.

A DEVELOPMENTAL VIEW OF EMOTIONS

Henry Krystal, an American psychoanalyst who has worked extensively with groups of patients suffering from intractable psychosomatic problems, such as survivors of Nazi concentration camps and drug addicts, has pointed out in his book *Integration and Self-Healing* that a developmental view of emotions contributes significantly to our understanding of psychosomatic illnesses and diseases and to finding appropriate ways of treating them (Krystal 1988).

In Krystal's view, all emotions attain their mature form after a lifelong development from *affect precursors*. The newborn baby experiences emotions as *internal tensions which are perceived as diffuse excitement on an undifferentiated sensorimotor level*. This very quickly becomes differentiated into two general types of affect precursor, one a state of contentment and the other of generalised distress. From the patterns of contentment and tranquillity develop the positive affects, and from the agitated states of discomfort and distress evolve the negative affects. The biological component of these primitive emotions is very strong and affects are experienced as physical sensations. At birth the affective display of the newborn is the only mode of non-verbal communication with the mother and affects are essentially signals for another person. As emotions mature they can become signals for the self. The idea of affects as signals conveying information is central to the idea of self-regulation, but initially the baby relies on the mother's tender holding and sensitive handling for regulation of emotional arousal.

The emotions mature along two developmental lines: *affect differentiation* and *affect verbalisation with concomitant de-somatisation*. In the process their biological components become less intense.

These affective developments take place within the facilitating environment provided by what Winnicott called 'a good enough mother' (Winnicott 1972). The development of language and symbolisation is the fundamental event in the development of affect symbolisation. As verbal skills and symbolisation develop, the precision and effectiveness of words demonstrate language to be the preferred way of handling affects. As the affect components mature and differentiate it becomes clear that the cognitive aspects of an emotion have a meaning and a story.

Robert Stoller, in *Observing the Erotic Imagination*, has given an example of how language can assist the differentiation of the experience of the affect Distress-Anguish, or sadness as it is commonly known, into finer nuances of meaning.

When we sense that we are sad, we have to try to identify whether we are very sad, regretfully sad, tragically sad, deeply sad, sad dreary, sad dull, sad troubled, sad strong, bitter sad, sad wretched, sad rueful, genuinely sad, glad to be sad, sad without grief, bravely sad, shallowly sad, noisily sad, choked up sad, tearfully sad, lachrymosely sad, whiningly sad, voluptuously sad, sad after a homosexual loss, sad after a heterosexual loss, sad after a heterosexual loss mitigated by unconscious homosexual relief, sad for a moment, sad for two days, sad anxious, sad guilty, sad as a mood to be in that always leads to erotic excitement, sad as a transference relationship, sad with a sad smile, sad yet amused, sad from an old memory, sad from a trashy song, elegiac, nostalgic, wistful, longing, yearning, sober, pitiful, miserable, bathetic, glum, broken hearted, forlorn, desolated, lugubrious, dolorous, woeful, despairing, dampened, crestfallen, blue, melancholic, gloomy, depressed rather than sad. (Stoller 1985)

The more precise the recognition of one's feelings, the greater their utility as a signal to the self, carrying information about the relationship to the self and to others and the more likely they are to contribute to the powers of self-monitoring and self-regulation.

It is the mature, adult, well regulated type of affects that are best suited for signal functions. Such affects are minimal in the intensity of their physiological components, are appropriate to the circumstances in which they arise and they are mainly cognitive and resemble ideas. It is important to emphasise that although the physiological component of well modulated emotion can become attenuated, it never entirely disappears, and it is normal for individuals to experience somatic sensations that accompany their emotional arousal. We may experience butterflies in our stomach before an interview or an examination, or aches and pains from increased muscle tension, but do not become alarmed because we have recognised the provoking stimulus and regard the somatic sensations as secondary phenomena. In excessive unregulated emotion, however, the subject may not recognise the provoking stimulus. He is particularly likely to ignore it if the stimulus is an internal, psychic one. If he fails to recognise it, he will not understand the bodily sensations that he experiences and is therefore likely to look upon them as primary phenomena; his fear about their possible medical significance dominates his consciousness. Sustained, unregulated, intense emotions can lead to disregulation of other biological systems in the body and becomes a risk factor for the development of disease.

AFFECT REGULATION AND SOME RELATED CONCEPTS: EMOTIONAL INTELLIGENCE, EMOTIONAL AWARENESS, SOLACE

If all goes well and the person is lucky enough to have been brought up by parents or carers who have held him empathically, he may reach a stage in his emotional development which is characterised by the emotional competencies that have recently been described as 'emotional intelligence'. This concept refers to the cognitive skills required to effectively monitor and self-regulate the emotions. It was first elaborated by Salovey, Hsee and Mayer (1993) and is derived from the theory of multiple intelligences developed by Howard Gardner (1983).

Daniel Goleman made the concept accessible to the public in his best-selling book, *Emotional Intelligence*, in which he identified a set of cognitive skills that are the result of an advanced state of emotional development (Goleman 1995).

These skills are characterised by the ability to recognise one's feelings, to distinguish between them, to regulate one's mood, to resist the impulse to express an emotion in action, to keep distress from swamping the capacity to think, to hope, to motivate oneself, to persist in the face of frustration and to understand other people's feelings.

Two more emotional skills should be added which although they are not included in the construct of emotional intelligence, are also very helpful in developing and maintaining mature and harmonious relationships.

One emotional skill, the ability to give credit to oneself, has been emphasised by Michael Basch in *Understanding Psychotherapy*. It relates to a resilient attributional style that allows the maintenance of a sense of self esteem and optimism even in adversity (Basch 1988).

The other is a sense of mature humour which is characterised by the fact that the joke is on oneself rather than on someone else and is referred to as one of the mature defences of the ego (Vaillant 1993).

Cognitive processes are not of course the only way of regulating emotions. The development of transitional phenomena and the capacity for imaginative play, as well as relationships characterised by secure attachment, are important contributors to affect regulation. Affects may also regulate other affects. The activation of positive emotions, such as interest or hope, counteracts negative ones such as fear or sadness and thereby alleviates a tendency to depression, whereas shame may attenuate joy. Play or other imaginative activity enhances the positive emotions of interest and enjoyment; these have regulatory feedback effects serving not only to minimise negative emotions but also to motivate further playful activity that intensifies interest.

Emotional Awareness

Lane and Schwartz, in a seminal paper (1987), propose that emotional awareness is the consequence of cognitive processing of emotional arousal, and that the cognitive process itself undergoes a sequence of structural transformations during development which, in turn, determines the structure of subsequent emotional experience.

They have described five levels of emotional awareness:

1. Awareness of bodily sensations only. At this level awareness of the separate existence of the other is minimal or non-existent.
2. Awareness of bodily sensations and action tendencies.
3. Awareness of individual feelings.
4. Awareness of blends of feelings.
5. Awareness of blends of blends of feelings.

At the fifth and highest level, the major advance is the development of empathy. The person can appreciate the experience of others in the context of an ongoing differentiated awareness of his own emotional experience. As a continuum construct, emotional intelligence corresponds to the higher levels of emotional awareness and is associated with the capacity to use emotions as signals to oneself and modulate emotional arousal. Individuals functioning at the lower levels can also be described as alexithymic.

AFFECT DISREGULATION AND SOME RELATED CONCEPTS: EMOTIONAL UNAWARENESS, AFFECT REGRESSION, INCONSOLABILITY, ALEXITHYMIA

A Clinical Example: George

George was sixty-nine years old when he started bleeding from the back passage for the first time in his life two weeks after his wife was diagnosed as suffering from carcinoma of the breast. I had known the couple for many years and they had always been very close. Although his wife became very distressed and frightened following the diagnosis, he seemed to be very calm and supportive. Soon she had the cancerous lump removed, and as there was no spread of the disease the prognosis was considered to be good.

However, George's bleeding became worse. He was investigated in hospital and it was found on bowel histology that he was suffering from Crohn's disease, which is a form of inflammatory bowel disease.

As his bleeding started so soon after the diagnosis of his wife's illness, I wondered whether his grief about the loss of his wife's health might have something to do with the onset of his disease. During a consultation, when I tried to explore his emotions and asked him whether it was possible that his wife's illness was getting him down, he looked at me with complete incomprehension. He replied that he had read somewhere that Crohn's disease can be caused by tightening the belt too hard. As he used to wear a tight corset for support of his back for many years, he wondered whether inadvertently he had damaged himself.

His answer confused me and put me off asking any more questions that day. With his reply I felt that he created a barrier to my effort to explore his emotional life.

However, I pursued the matter at another session and gradually it emerged that he did not understand what I meant by stress. He did not experience any mental anguish. He did not feel worried, sad, depressed or frightened about the future of his relationship to his wife. The only thing that he felt sad about was that due to his rectal bleeding he could not go out and about in the West End as he used to. He had a very stoic attitude, saying more or less that life has its ups and downs and one must accept both with equanimity. A few days after our conversation his disease deteriorated dramatically and a large part of his bowel had to be removed surgically. He developed post-operative complications and he was admitted to the intensive care unit where he died six weeks later.

Emotional Unawareness

When I tried to have a conversation with George about his feelings, I was hoping that by sharing his negative emotions I would help him modulate their intensity and make them more tolerable. I was therefore shocked to discover the discrepancy between the feelings I imagined he would have about his wife's illness and the feelings he actually had. When we are empathic and put ourselves in our patients' shoes, trying to imagine the kind of feelings they must be experiencing, we are assuming that everyone will have the same emotions under similar circumstances and that a named emotion always refers to the exact duplicate of our own. This is a very adaptive assumption which most of the time confirms our common humanity. However, the above case illustrates that this assumption cannot be taken for granted, and that the patient's style of experiencing and communicating emotions has to be identified and taken into account.

The rectal bleeding occurred at a time when I would have expected the patient to experience certain intense feelings, but he did not. Why not? What happened to his feelings? Very often we use the word 'denial' to explain this ignoring of emotional reality, but somehow the term does not seem adequate to describe what appears to be a much more radical difficulty at the level of processing emotions. Terms such as 'dissociation', 'disavowal', 'emotional unawareness', 'foreclosure of emotions from the psyche', 'lack of psychological-mindedness', 'emotional illiteracy', and 'alexithymia' have been used by researchers in an attempt to describe this apparent absence of feelings. All these personality characteristics are related and interfere with the cognitive processing of affects that can lead to modulation of the intensity of their physiological components.

Alexithymia

Graeme Taylor has given a full account of the development of the concept of alexithymia which can be thought of as being the opposite of emotional intelligence (Taylor and Bagby 1999).

The concept was coined by an American psychiatrist of Greek origins, Peter Sifneos (1973), who, with Nemiah in the early 1970s, began to investigate systematically the cognitive and affective style of patients suffering from psychosomatic diseases. They found that sixteen out of the twenty patients they studied showed a marked difficulty in verbally expressing or describing their feelings, had an impoverished fantasy life and a cognitive style that was literal, utilitarian and externally oriented.

Similar observations had been made before, by Ruesch (1948) and MacLean (1949) who speculated that upsetting emotions find immediate expression through the autonomic pathways and are translated into organ language instead of being relayed to the neocortex and finding expression in the symbolic use of words.

It was Sifneos's strikingly apt choice of the word 'alexithymia' that captured the essence of this particular communicative style. Alexithymia is in fact a neologism and is made up from the Greek: *a* – lack, *lexis* – word, *thymos* – emotion. Literally, 'no words for emotions'. However, we must not accept the literal translation of the word 'alexithymia' because alexithymic patients do have an emotional vocabulary, albeit a limited one. They may complain of depression or anxiety or stress, but if they are asked to elaborate on their feelings they will talk about somatic sensations mainly.

Marty and de M'Uzan (1963) in France used the term *pensée opératoire* to describe a similar utilitarian cognitive style among physically ill patients.

Quite independently, but in parallel to Sifneos's work, Henry Krystal was reporting similar characteristics in patients with post-traumatic states. The traumatic origin of alexithymia was also emphasised by Wurmser (1994) who attributed it to the global denial of traumatically intense feelings, caused by an underlying intense shame.

The concept of alexithymia generated a lot of research and debate among psychosomatic doctors, and in 1976 at the 11th European conference on psychosomatic research in Heidelberg, it was concluded that clinicians and researchers should agree upon a precise formulation and definition of the alexithymia construct.

Following the conference the most enduring features of alexithymia were found to be:

1. Difficulty in identifying and naming emotions and describing them to other people.
2. Difficulty distinguishing between feelings and bodily sensations of emotional arousal.
3. That the thinking of alexithymic persons has a utilitarian style, concentrating on environmental detail and showing a striking absence of fantasies and imagination.

Over the past decade measurement-based and experimental studies have yielded considerable empirical support for the alexithymia construct. In addition the development of the Toronto Alexithymia Scale (TAS) and the revised Twenty-Item Toronto Alexithymia Scale (TAS-20) provided reliable and valid methods for measuring the construct. These self-report scales have been cross-validated in diverse cultures and are now the most widely used measures of alexithymia.

Alexithymia therefore represents a deficit in cognitive processing and experiencing of emotions which has an important role to play in the regulation of emotional arousal.

In a recent paper, Taylor reviewed the possible pathways whereby the associated disregulation could influence bodily processes (Taylor 2000). These include unhealthy behaviours often associated with alexithymia, such as substance abuse or disordered eating, as well as sustained arousal of the physiological component of the emotion response. Although knowledge of the physiological correlates of alexithymia is currently inconclusive, some of the somatic disorders that coincide with high rates of alexithymia are known to be associated with sympatho-vagal imbalance. Essential hypertension for example, has been linked not only with heightened sympathetic activity but also with reduced vagal tone (Langewitz et al. 1994). Some researchers have suggested that the association between alexithymia and morbidity may be due to the effects of alexithymia on the patients' verbal communication of emotional distress to their carers and doctors. This is so poor that they fail to enlist others for help or comfort. Others have found evidence that alexithymia can have a negative influence on the quality of life in patients with chronic disease. After many years of research on alexithymia the alexithymic communicative style is no longer thought to be specific to patients with classical psychosomatic diseases, but is now regarded as one of several possible situations of general onset, or risk factors, that seem to increase susceptibility to disease specified by other variables. Furthermore, because symbolic communication is limited, alexithymia has been described as possibly the most important single factor that diminishes the success of psychoanalysis and psychodynamic psychotherapy.

CONCLUSION

Recent research has demonstrated that contrasting the irrationality of emotions to the rationality of reasoning and decision-making is no longer tenable. The structures of the brain responsible for emotional processing are an integral part of the neural machinery of reason. Their damage leads to flawed reasoning (Damasio 1996). At present emotions are viewed as multifaceted phenomena which are simultaneously somatic and psychological, and therefore bridge the mind–body divide. They are understood as an evolutionary extension of homoeostasis which means that in the disregulation model of psychosomatic medicine they are viewed as an important signalling system that contributes to the regulation of the behaviour of the organism and of its components. Emotions not only produce somatic sensations that can be misinterpreted as symptoms of physical disease and responded to maladaptively, but also, in the presence of deficits in emotional processing and regulation, may become risk factors for the development of disease by leading to disregulation of other biological systems.

4 EMOTIONS AND IMMUNITY: THE EMOTIONAL CONTEXT PRECEDING THE ERUPTION OF HERPES ZOSTER

WHAT IS HERPES ZOSTER?

Two words are used to describe this disease: zoster and shingles. Zoster is a Greek word meaning girdle, and shingles, according to the *Oxford English Dictionary*, is a mediaeval English word deriving from the Latin *cingulum*, meaning the same thing. This is a graphic description of the linear blistery rash of the disease, which always occurs on one side of the body and usually affects the waist area like a blister-studded belt.

As every doctor knows, herpes zoster is an infection of the peripheral nervous system and is caused by the reactivation of the varicella zoster virus (VZV) which also causes chickenpox when the person, usually in childhood, is initially exposed to it. As the immune system mounts its response to bring the chickenpox under control, the virus migrates inwards along the sensory nerves and reaches the dorsal root ganglia which are situated alongside the spinal cord and the trigeminal ganglia inside the skull, where it remains dormant for the rest of the person's life. The exact biological mechanisms that keep the virus in latent form are not known, but cellular immunity, which involves the T-lymphocytes, macrophages and Natural Killer Cells, is very important.

When the control exercised by the cellular immunity falters, the virus is reactivated and starts replicating. It progresses peripherally down the sensory nerve to produce the typical blistery rash which is restricted to the area of the skin supplied by that nerve, known as a dermatome. When the rash occupies the whole dermatome there is no doubt about the diagnosis. When, however, the rash involves a small cluster of blisters, it is impossible to know without serological tests whether we are dealing with partially expressed VZV, or infection with the related virus herpes simplex, which can cause a similar rash. The last two patients of my series of ten did not have a dermatomal rash but their experience of stress was similar to those who had herpes zoster. Although rarely a life-threatening disease, herpes zoster is of concern because of the pain it can cause and the risk of developing neuralgia following the acute lesion. This post-herpetic neuralgia is defined as the persistence of pain beyond healing of the acute lesion. Because the natural history of herpetic neuralgia is gradual resolution of pain after the vesicles heal, the point at which the acute condition is termed post-herpetic is a matter of definition. A reasonable definition considers post-herpetic neuralgia to be pain persisting for longer than two months after healing of the vesicles.

Overall 12–20 per cent of patients with the acute condition complain of pain after the vesicles heal. This figure drops to 9 per cent at four weeks and to 1–2 per cent at one year. The rates are greatly affected by age, however, and in one large survey pain persisted for more than one year in 50 per cent of patients aged seventy or more. Post-herpetic neuralgia typically has several components including constant burning, lancinating pain, deep aching and allodynia, which means pain induced by non-painful stimuli such as stroking. Commonly associated with pain are depressed mood, sleep disturbance, anorexia and weight loss (Galer and Portenoy 1991).

THE DEVELOPMENT OF MY INTEREST

It is well known among hospital doctors that shingles occurs more frequently in the immunosuppressed, such as those who receive chemotherapy for a malignancy, AIDS sufferers and the elderly. However, the majority of patients with shingles who present at my surgery in Hackney are healthy and middle-aged. Since I became a partner at the Well Street Surgery in December 1986, I have recorded every consultation with shingles patients. In my first nine years in general practice I saw thirty-eight patients. Their mean age was forty-five and none had a medical explanation for immuno-suppression.

What was going on? What could be causing immunosuppression of equivalent severity to cancer or AIDS, which was sufficient to allow for the development of disease? At the beginning of my general practice career, a good friend had developed shingles a few weeks before his wedding and I realised then that the eruption of herpes zoster might not be a random event. At about the same time Dr John Paulley, one of the pioneers in psychoso-matic medicine in England, introduced me to the work of Bartrop who, in 1977, found that the responsiveness of T-lymphocytes taken from bereaved people was significantly reduced when compared to the responsiveness of T-lymphocytes from people who had not been bereaved. I wondered therefore whether loss or other stresses might be responsible for the immunosuppres-sion. Certainly, listening to my patients' stories I had formed the impression that all of them were very stressed before shingles erupted and most of them were reticent in talking about their distress. I thought at the time that their reticence was due to lack of awareness of their emotional distress and that this was a manifestation of alexithymia.

In 1995 Lesley Southgate who was then working at our surgery and was also professor of general practice at St. Bartholomew's Hospital invited local general practitioners to become research associates in her department and develop protocols for research projects to test their ideas. She already knew of my observations regarding the importance of stress in the eruption of shingles and she encouraged me to formulate a research proposal and participate in her scheme. As I had great admiration for Dr Peter White's psychosomatic research on chronic fatigue, I asked his advice as to whether my idea that stress and alexithymia might be risk factors for shingles could be tested. He thought that it could and he introduced me to Tirril Harris who had devised a method for measuring stress by grading the severity of life events and difficulties. The next step was to choose a study design that could realistically be carried out with the very limited resources available to me in the general practice setting. Dr Chris Griffiths, my tutor, a senior lecturer at the department of general practice who was experienced in research methodology, helped me to construct a case control study that would compare the intensity of stressful experiences and the degree of alexithymia of patients who developed shingles with those of a control group, such as patients who developed ringworm, a fungal infection of the skin where stress is not thought to be important.

WHAT IS STRESS?

It is far more acceptable to people to talk about the impersonal concept of stress rather than their emotions. It may be that in part the word owes its acceptability to a certain ambiguity, because stress is a term that refers both to the stressor and to the ensuing distress. Further confusion arises because the same word is loosely used to indicate any form of emotional unease, ranging from the effort needed to solve a mathematical problem to the ravages of bereavement or a nuclear disaster.

The most widely accepted definitions of stress focus on the individual's inability to meet environmental demands and the negative emotions of hopelessness and helplessness that occur when a situation threatens to exceed the capacity to deal with it. Life events are stressors and they contribute to an increased predisposition to disease through the activation of emotional distress and maladaptive behaviours. Distress is another ambiguous word that refers both to the arousal of non-specific negative emotions and the particular strategies that people have to manage them. For instance, some people show their distress by getting drunk, smoking excessively, eating too much, and so on. It must not be confused with the way Tomkins uses the word 'distress' to indicate the low end of the spectrum of sadness (Tomkins 1963). William Miller, a professor of law at the University of Michigan Law School, who has written extensively on the emotions of humiliation and disgust, points out that the word 'distress', in the imprecise sense of negative emotions, is a homage we pay to the fact that we rarely experience one emotion unaccompanied by others. Emotions flood in upon us as we respond emotionally to our own emotional states. We are guilty about our anger, disgusted by our fear, embarrassed by our grief, furious about our humiliation (Miller 1997). Donald Nathanson understands the term 'stress' to refer to the upper range of affective experience which occurs when the experiencing of several negative emotions together, one amplifying the other, produces sequences of terrible vehemence, so that we lose the ability to name each affect separately (Nathanson 1992). Unfortunately the strategies that most people have to deal with the toxic experience of negative affect do not always induce calm. The ability to adaptively modulate the affective response is essential for the mastery of stress and in clinical work this is one of my primary considerations

HOW DO WE MEASURE STRESS?

One of the best ways to measure stress at present is with the Life Events and Difficulties Schedule (LEDS). This is a semi-structured interview developed and validated by Tirril Harris, George Brown and other researchers at the Bedford Square College during their research on the social origins of depression (Brown and Harris 1978, 1981).

As the success of this instrument depends on the skill of the interviewer, I had first to train to use it in a course ran by Harris.

Because herpes zoster is an acute disease, Tirril Harris advised me to concentrate my investigation on the year preceding the eruption of shingles and also to use a measure of depression, the Beck Depression Inventory (BDI) (Beck et al. 1961).

Life events are stressors and contribute to an increased predisposition to disease through the activation of negative emotions and maladaptive behaviours. In the psychosomatic model that informs my research, however, increased susceptibility to disease requires an interaction between emotionally stressful life events and a personality predisposition. Examples of personality predispositions to disease are such constructs as alexithymia, hostility, and Type C behaviour pattern.

Alexithymia, as previously explained, describes a personality trait characterised by difficulty in expressing feelings verbally and an absence of a rich fantasy life. Graeme Taylor and his collaborators have devised and validated a questionnaire, the Toronto Alexithymia Scale (TAS-20)* that can identify persons with this particular communicative style (Taylor 1994).

Hostility is the component of Type A behaviour pattern that has been found recently to be a risk factor for the development of ischaemic heart disease and other diseases, such as peptic ulcers, asthma, rheumatoid arthritis and thyroid problems. Three aspects of hostility are especially harmful to health. Cynicism: a mistrusting attitude regarding the motives of people in general, leading one to be constantly on guard against the misbehaviour of others. Anger: the emotion so often engendered by the cynical person's expectation of unacceptable behaviour on the part of others. Aggression: the behaviour to which many hostile people are driven by the

---

* More information about using the Toronto Alexithymia Scale (TAS-20) can be obtained from Professor Taylor's website: <http://www.gtaylorpsychiatry.org>

unpleasant negative emotion of anger, irritation and the like (Williams and Williams 1994).

The Type C behaviour pattern is characterised by suppressing one's needs and feelings and harbouring chronic feelings of hopelessness hidden behind a mask of normality, until this defensive style is overwhelmed by an accumulation of stressful life events. Lydia Temoshok (1985) operationalised the construct of Type C behaviour pattern and found that it correlated significantly with the thickness of the initial skin lesions of malignant melanomas (Temoshok et al. 1985).

THE PATTERN OF EMOTIONS PRECEDING THE ERUPTION OF HERPES ZOSTER

The collection of information with the LEDS is fairly laborious. With the patient's permission I tape-record the interview, which may last from one to five hours depending on how much the patient has to say; indeed, it may spread over several days. Listening to it again, I arrange the information scattered throughout the tape into distinct life events and difficulties and then present them to a consensus meeting led by Tirril Harris and whose members rate each event and difficulty according to the perceived degree of threat or unpleasantness for the patient. The ratings are expressed numerically and can be manipulated mathematically and compared with those of controls. To avoid bias in these ratings by the members of the group, I deliberately do not tell them what type of rash each patient is suffering. Because LEDS surveys every aspect of a patient's life in a systematic way, I began to collect information that was beyond the scope of ordinary general practice consultations. From the first few interviews I realised that the pattern of narratives of the patients who developed shingles had in common a powerful and persuasive consistency which they did not share with the controls. This chapter is based on this research and focuses only on the narratives of patients who developed shingles, constructed from the information gathered using the semi-structured interview.

The pattern had three components:

1. An event or incident that aroused strong feelings of anger or fear or both, between one and seven days before the eruption of shingles.
2. Ongoing difficulties that aroused a blend of chronic negative emotions over several months before the eruption.
3. Frequent experience of early loss or adversity that provided a reservoir of non-declarative, fear memories which created bodily changes when these were retrieved.

Contrary to expectations, only one of the patients, Scott, was alexithymic, and only two of the ten patients, Rita and Winnie, had BDI scores in the range of mild depression. The rest had minimal scores. So it seems that alexithymia and depression will turn out not to be significant risk factors for the eruption of shingles. None of the patients I have seen so far has developed post herpetic neuralgia.

Only one published paper investigates whether life events are risk factors for herpes zoster. Kenneth Schmader and his colleagues (1990) concluded that whereas patients with herpes zoster experienced the same kinds of life events in the year preceding the disease as did control subjects, recent events perceived as stressful were significantly more common among patients with zoster. Thus stressful life events may be a risk factor for the reactivation of VZV. Their subjects, however, were aged over fifty. They also used the Geriatric Scale of Recent Life Events, which is a modification of the Social Readjustment Ratings Scale (Holmes and Rahe 1967). The data were collected by an expert telephone interviewer who was aware of 'case' and 'control' status but was not aware of the study hypothesis. Consent to participate in the research was obtained from 101 patients with shingles who were included in the study. The same number of controls were located by random digit dialling (Schmader et al. 1990).

TOWARDS SOLVING THE MYSTERY OF THE LEAP FROM THE MIND TO THE BODY

Although I have come to the conclusion that emotions are an important factor in the eruption of shingles, there is still a challenge in trying to explain how intangible feelings can give rise to tangible bodily changes such as the blistery rash of herpes zoster. Paul Martin, in his book *The Sickening Mind*, finds that the answer to this problem became possible in 1970 when Robert Ader, a psychologist, and Nicholas Cohen, an immunologist, discovered that the immune system (IS) and the central nervous system (CNS) communicate (Martin 1997). Theirs was a serendipitous discovery. Ader and Cohen were studying a form of behavioural conditioning known as learned taste aversion. As part of their research they conditioned rats by giving them saccharine-sweetened water along with cyclophosphamide, a drug that causes nausea and suppresses the immune system, and in particular the T-lymphocytes. Soon the rats learned, through Pavlovian conditioning, to avoid sweet water because they associated it with the nausea. Ader discovered, however, that after a certain time, giving the rats saccharine-sweetened water alone, without the cytotoxic drug, still resulted in a lowering of their T-cell count to the point that some rats began dying of infectious diseases. This was puzzling. How was it possible for an immunologically neutral stimulus like sweetness to make a rat die? The investigators hypothesised that conditioning might have caused the previously neutral stimulus, the sweet taste, to elicit the same biological response as the drug, namely immune suppression. They put their hypothesis to the test by injecting the immune conditioned rats with red cells taken from sheep which are a powerful antigen. They found that the rats that had been subjected to immune conditioning produced significantly fewer antibodies. The sweet taste itself was sufficient to reduce the antibody response by a quarter. This meant that the immune system like the CNS could learn. It is difficult for us today to imagine the sense of shock that the scientific community experienced at the time. Until that day every doctor, every biologist, every physiologist, every immunologist, considered the immune system to be an autonomous entity that operated to a large degree with no regard to the integrated physiology of the organism. Until then, no pathways were known to connect the rat brain centres that monitor taste with parts of the immune system responsible for the immune response. This discovery marked the beginning of a new field of research called psychoneuroimmunology which studies how the parts of the brain responsible for emotions and the immune system influence each other (Ader et al. 1995). Michel Odent (1999) has coined the term 'primal adaptive system' to refer to this very complex psychoneuroimmunoendocrinological network. The term 'primal' (first in time and first in importance) stresses that this network reaches a high degree of maturity as early as during the 'primal period', that is from conception until the first birthday.

MEMORIES OF EARLY LOSS AND ADVERSITY

Cathy, the ninth patient in my series of ten, is a very good example of the biological effects that retrieval of an emotional memory can have on the body. In order to appreciate the biological significance of memories of early loss and adversity, it is important to discuss briefly the distinction between explicit, declarative or narrative memories which can be brought to mind and described verbally, and implicit non-declarative memories created through the mechanism of fear conditioning.

Modern studies of the brain mechanisms of memory have demonstrated that there are two different memory systems. One is involved in forming memories of experiences and making these available to conscious recollection, which are referred to as declarative or narrative memories. The hippocampal circuits with their massive neocortical interconnections are the main components of this system. Another is operating outside consciousness and controlling behaviour without explicit awareness of past learning. This system forms implicit, or non-declarative memories about dangerous or otherwise threatening situations in which the amygdala is the key anatomical structure. Memories of this type are created through the mechanisms of fear conditioning. The learning that occurs does not depend on conscious awareness and, once the learning has taken place, the stimulus need not be consciously perceived in order to elicit the conditioned emotional response.

Joseph Le Doux, in *The Emotional Brain* (1998), gives a simple example that makes it easy to understand how the two memory systems operate.

Suppose that you are driving down the road and have a terrible accident. The horn cannot be turned off, you are in pain and generally traumatised by the experience. Later when you hear the sound of a horn both the implicit and explicit memory systems are activated. The sound of the horn having become a conditioned fear stimulus, goes straight from the auditory system, through the thalamus to the amygdala bypassing the auditory cortex and implicitly elicits bodily responses that typically occur in situations of danger such as increased muscle tension (a vestige of freezing with fear), changes in blood pressure and heart rate, changes in breathing pattern, increased perspiration, immune changes and so on. The sound also travels through the cortex to the temporal lobe memory system where explicit declarative memories are activated. You are reminded of the accident, you consciously remember how awful it was, but the declarative memory system does not involve actual bodily changes, but only that you were injured and that the accident was awful. These facts are propositions that can be declared about the experience. The particular fact that the accident was awful is not emotional memory. It is a declarative memory about an emotional experience. It is mediated by the temporal lobe memory system and has no biological consequences. In order to have an aversive emotional memory complete with the bodily experiences that come with an emotion, you have to activate an emotional memory system such as that of the implicit fear memory system involving the amygdala.

For example, suppose that the accident described above happened long ago and your explicit memory system has since then forgotten many of the details, such as the fact that the horn had been stuck on. The sound of the horn now, many years later, is ignored by the explicit memory system. But the emotional memory system has not forgotten. The sound of the horn when it reaches the amygdala will trigger an emotional reaction with all its physiological activation. In a situation like this you find yourself in the throes of an emotional state that exists for reasons you do not understand. In order for emotion to be aroused in this way the implicit emotional memory system would have to be less forgetful than the explicit memory system. Indeed, recent research has demonstrated that this is the case. Conditioned fear responses not only do not diminish with time but often increase their potency as time wears on, a phenomenon known as the incubation of fear. (Le Doux 1998)

There are two amygdala in the brain, one in each hemisphere and they are part of the old brain. Each amygdala is an almond-shaped cluster of interconnected structures situated above the brain stem and, as Le Doux discovered recently, they are the essential brain structures involved in the appraisal of the emotional meaning of stimuli. It is possible that implicitly processed stimuli activate the amygdala without activating explicit memories or otherwise being represented in consciousness.

Henry Krystal, an American psychoanalyst who has worked extensively with survivors of Nazi concentration camps and with drug addicts, both of whom suffer from intractable psychosomatic illnesses, has pointed out that because the acquisition of language and symbolisation is a gradual one, subject to lapse and distortion, many infantile memories have to be viewed as non-symbolic, non-verbalisable affect memories. When these primitive, pre-verbal, non-declarative memories are retrieved, their somatic component is very strong and the person is not aware of their precise nature. They are felt at a sensory motor level of emotional awareness and experienced as physical symptoms contributing to emotional disregulation (Krystal 1988).

The existence of separate systems for storing implicit emotional memories and explicit memories of emotions helps us understand how the content of memory is influenced by emotional states. Learning that takes place in one emotional state is generally best remembered when we are in a similar state.

STORIES OF SHINGLES

Rita

Rita is a seventy-three-year-old woman; tall, well built, with short grey hair, who speaks with a heavy Italian accent and is always apologetic when she comes to tell me of her various complaints.

Shingles

One day she presented with a T5 dermatomal herpes zoster rash, extending from the sternum, over her mastectomy scar to her axilla and all the way round to her spine. Although the rash was extensive, the blisters were not very dense and formed two large clusters, one at the front and the other at the back, with a few scattered blisters in between.

Rita lives in a council maisonette with her husband Carlo who is the same age as her. They have three grown-up children.

Ongoing Stress

Rita met Carlo in her twenties when she was working as a waitress and fell in love with his dapper looks. Her parents opposed her marriage and her father disinherited her rather than let Carlo benefit from his money. They came to London where Carlo worked as a motor mechanic and she found work as a domestic in a hospital. It had not been easy being married to Carlo. He is an aggressive man, unsociable and a loner. When he came home from work he used to demand angrily to have his dinner immediately and he did not like having the children around. He used to hit the children and on several occasions he gave Rita a black eye. She did not imagine he would be like this when she married him. He has never been interested in other women and he has never been unfaithful, but he has not been very interested in her either. When she needed to have a hysterectomy because of abnormal bleeding he would not give his consent as next of kin, and when she developed cancer of the breast and needed to have a mastectomy he did not want her to have one. In fact their sexual life ended after her mastectomy fifteen years ago. She has never slept with him since then. Carlo had always been a heavy smoker and he developed ischaemic heart disease. *Five months before the eruption* of her shingles he had heart surgery following a myocardial infarction, and although his breathing improved after the operation, he has not stopped moaning and smoking. He sits upstairs watching TV all day long and chain-smokes. When she reminds him that smoking will harm his heart, he replies that he has nothing else in life and he does not care. Although Rita is suffering from chronic bronchitis and heart failure and her doctors have advised her not to inhale smoke, he does not care about her health either and refuses to stop smoking. Rita has come to the surgery many times complaining of a persistent productive cough which is not responding to any medication. Carlo has been more aggressive than ever since his operation. He shouts and swears at her and keeps telling her that she is a lousy cook and that she is always ill and moaning. He has stopped hitting her, however. Rita says that if he tried to hit her now she would push him downstairs. She has had enough. Her children wanted her to leave him long ago but she is old-fashioned and believes that you marry for better or worse. You have to grin and bear it.

Rita had been concerned about her eldest daughter Donna who, after divorcing her husband, was in the process of selling her marital home. *Eight months before the eruption* of Rita's shingles Donna had a hysterectomy for abnormal bleeding and like Rita she had suffered bladder damage. She lives in another city and since her operation she had been telephoning her mother frequently and complaining of breast pain.

Acute Fear of her Daughter's Phone Call

Rita finally persuaded her to ask for a mammogram from her doctor, and *one day before the eruption*, Donna rang her mother in tears. She was very frightened because she had received a letter asking her to go back to the hospital for more tests. Rita remained calm during the telephone conversation and managed to reassure her daughter, but as soon as she put the receiver down she burst into tears and cried for a long time inconsolably. She was very worried about Donna's health because their medical histories had been identical so far with the hysterectomy and bladder complications and it was possible that Donna might develop the breast cancer too. She cried because she felt that Donna's problems were all her fault. She was very unhappy when she was pregnant with Donna because of her husband who would not find a job and who was cruel to her and she believed that if a pregnant mother is unhappy then the child she carries becomes depressed, and that this unhappiness has something to do with the breast cancer. Also, she could understand how frightened Donna must have been because she remembered her own fear when she was told she had breast cancer. She said that the night after that phone call she felt 'anyhow' and she could not sleep. When she got up in the morning she noticed the blistery rash of shingles.

Thomas

Thomas is a fifty-year-old accountant, who came to London twenty years ago as a political refugee from Poland with his wife Sarah, one year after they had been released from prison. He is a stockily built man who has a gentle, thoughtful expression and speaks softly with a pleasant, faint accent.

Shingles

One day he experienced pain in his right loin. The following day he developed a group of blisters in a small area the size of a 50p coin, and went to see his doctor. Two days later the blisters spread and the rash was very dense. In another four days the blisters had coalesced and extended round his waist and had occupied the whole area of the T10 dermatome when he came to see me. The area of the rash was covered in a yellow crust, and as he had a high temperature I presumed that the rash was superinfected with staphylococci, and so I treated him with a combination of antibacterial and antiviral antibiotics. His pain was intense and he needed painkillers every two hours.

Ongoing Stress

Although Thomas had a university degree, he did not speak a word of English when he came to Britain. He was obliged to do a variety of odd jobs while he was learning the language. For the last ten years he had been working as an accountant in a large firm, and over the last two years he experienced a doubling of the amount of work. The company had grown, the demand had increased and he felt he could not always work to the high standard he expected of himself. He was fed up with his job and he would prefer to be a sales representative for a winery, promoting the beautiful wines of his country.

Thomas had met Sarah at university. They love each other, they have the same interests and they enjoy their conversation. She is his confidante. Soon after they came to England they had a son, but around the same time she developed asthma which has gradually been getting worse. Because she gets breathless climbing the stairs, they had to move their bed to the ground floor. Her breathing difficulty is putting him off sex, but that does not mean that they love each other any less. Sarah can become very breathless very fast and then she requires steroids and nebulised medication. When Thomas sees her having an asthmatic attack he feels dreadful because he feels powerless to make her better. He calls the doctor, tries to calm her down and reassures her that the doctor is on the way. Thomas's dream is to be able to return to his own country one day, but recently, with the deterioration of his wife's asthma, he has begun to fear that this dream may never come true. Medical care is very expensive in their country and not as readily available as in London, and he is afraid that Sarah will not get the prompt response to her asthmatic attacks that she has here and her life might be at risk. Because Sarah feels guilty about taking time off work she delays seeking medical attention until her asthma is extreme and she needs urgent hospital treatment. *Four months before the eruption* of his shingles she became so breathless that she became blue. She was rushed to hospital where the doctor told her that she nearly died because she did not take her illness seriously.

Thomas feels that if Sarah dies it will be the end of them as a family. She is the home-maker, and without her life in London will be intolerable. He will have to pack his things and go back to his country and he doubts whether he will be able to adjust to life there after so many years in England. He feels sad for her because she cannot enjoy life. His son is growing up and will leave home soon and Sarah is becoming incapacitated at a time when they could start enjoying life.

One month before the eruption of shingles Thomas's father died and he was buried within forty-eight hours. He could not go to the funeral because he was applying for British citizenship at the time and had sent his passport to the Home Office. The last time he had seen his father, six months previously, he had been making good progress from the stroke he had suffered a year earlier. Thomas felt very sad. He had known his father as a child and as a young man but not as an adult. When Thomas was arrested in his country he was only twenty-seven years old. He was released two years later and emigrated the following year. So he felt that in his adulthood he had been deprived of the opportunity to have a man to man relationship with his father. He always hoped that he could go back to his country and be able to enjoy the company of his father, his mother, his brothers and sisters. Now he worries about his elderly mother who lives alone. He tries to keep his worrying under control. He feels that he can switch off. He goes to work and forgets about it. He considers himself a cheerful person. He might get a little more irritable than usual and a little less sociable, but he manages to switch off. However, he often wakes up in the middle of the night and thinks and then he feels tired the next day.

Acute Fear on Hearing of his Sister's Illness

Two days before the shingles erupted his niece rang from Italy to say that her mother, Thomas's eldest sister, had been found to have a brain tumour. She had been complaining of headaches for some time and had consulted an optician who advised her to have a brain scan. The scan showed a brain tumour and the doctor recommended an immediate operation. Unfortunately the doctors were on strike and the operation could not be done immediately. She had had to wait for a week.

Thomas thought that the tumour must have been malignant if the doctor had recommended an immediate operation and felt very sorry for his sister. She was a schoolteacher who emigrated with her husband one year before Thomas. Her husband died of cancer three years later and she brought up her children alone. Recently she had become a grandmother and was looking forward to this fulfilling experience. Thomas felt close to her. He used to visit her often and kept in touch regularly by telephone. He felt very sad at the thought that the members of his family are reaching a critical age in their fifties and sixties and have started dying of dreadful diseases. He feared that his wife will be the next to go.

Thomas is unable to cry. He did not cry when his father died nor when he received the news about his sister. He admits that sometimes when he watches a 'silly' film his eyes water, but this is all. He feels sad, but he cannot cry even though he would like to. Unfortunately his sister died during the operation a week later, despite the eminence of the surgeon. His shingles gradually got worse in the week leading up to her operation and death so that he was unfit to travel to Italy for her funeral. Sarah went by herself and she had a severe asthmatic attack as soon as she returned.

Phil

Phil is a sixteen-year-old schoolboy who is tall and slim and probably too streetwise for his age.

Shingles

One day he developed a cluster of blisters at the tip of his right scapula the size of a 50p coin, and several more blisters, scattered between his scapula and spine, corresponding to dermatome T1.

Background

He lives with his mother, father, his twin brother, his older brother and foster brother in a large three-storey house which allows each one of them to have his own room. He is very close to his mother and his twin brother who are his confidants.

Ongoing Stress

One year before the eruption of shingles his twin brother developed pneumonia and became so breathless that Phil and his older brother had to carry him to the hospital where he remained for three weeks. This was a traumatic experience for Phil because he was afraid that his twin brother might die.

Seven months before the eruption of shingles his grandmother died. Her death was unexpected. His mother was very upset and was crying all the time. He tried hard to hold it all in, to be brave and not to cry. At the funeral he found it very hard trying to comfort his mother and keep a stiff upper lip.

Phil sees himself as the conciliator who is holding the whole family together. His foster brother, who is the same age as his older brother, is schiz-ophrenic, speaks with a Jamaican accent, smokes hash and gets £100 a week in invalidity benefit. His older brother is envious of his foster brother because he only gets £50 every two weeks in unemployment benefit. *Six months before the eruption of shingles* his older brother got drunk and had an argument with the foster brother. When his mother told him off, he flew off the handle and started smashing the house up and breaking the bathroom windows. Phil, who was in his own room with his mates at the time, pushed his older brother out of the house and prevented him from causing any more damage. It was a good thing that his father was not at home because there would have been a fight.

Phil is earning about £100 a week by doing a variety of jobs. He wakes up early and before he goes to school he goes to the local street market where he works for an hour helping a street trader to set up his stall. After school he goes back to the market and works for another two hours helping another street trader to pack his vegetables away. On Saturdays he works at the market for about ten hours helping several traders. He has been helping street traders since he was expelled from his secondary school, two years before the eruption of his shingles, because he was being rude to teachers, fighting with his fellow pupils and getting into arguments. The teachers kept a record of all his misdemeanours and compiled a booklet of all wrongdoings. It was horrible.

He had not always been the conciliator, but used to be quite a handful at home. He was out every night regardless of what his mum and dad said. However, being expelled from school was the best thing that could have happened to him. It had made him more open-minded and had made him think about why he had been thrown out. He thought about how to deal with situations and how not to get aggressive and throw his weight around. He found out that being quiet and minding his own business helped him cope with things better. He started going to a rehabilitation centre for three hours a day, and with the encouragement of his parents he started preparing to go back to school.

Six months before the eruption of his shingles he was enrolled in a new secondary school and started a new term. Suddenly, from working in his own time at a leisurely pace, he had a lot of deadlines to meet for essays, assignments and GCSE course work, and he found all this very stressful. Getting all this work done is very hard and there is not a day in the week that he does not think, 'God, I have to do this'; 'God, I have to do that.' Sometimes he leaves his work until the next day and the teacher demands the work and then he has to stay up until early morning trying to finish it in order to deliver it the next day. He has begun to regret being expelled from school. If he had held it all together he would not have had this break in his education which has left him ill-prepared to face present demands.

Acute Anger at Losing his Assignment

One day before the eruption of shingles, because he was behind with the delivery of an essay, his mum's friend was helping him to write it directly on the computer in order to save time. When he tried to save it, he pressed the wrong button and the essay was deleted. He could not believe it. He had spent five hours working for nothing. This was a complete let-down and he was very annoyed. He felt like kicking the computer, but he did not dare do it in front of his mother's friend. If she had not been there he would have kicked the computer clean off the table, but he had to hold it down. He groaned as he struggled to control the impulse to lash out violently. Fortunately, his mum's friend was very comforting. She told him not to worry and she would help him to do it all over again. The following day as he was playing football his back started aching and itching and he thought that he had been stung by a bee. When he looked at his back later that day he was surprised that the bite was so big.

Scott

Scott is a twenty-seven-year-old computer expert who works full time in the technical support department of a computer company.

Shingles

One day he woke up feeling very tired, as if he had run a marathon, and noticed that he had a small group of blisters under his left nipple. When he came to see me five days later, the rash had spread to occupy the whole of the T7 dermatome, extending from his sternum round his axilla to his spine. A cluster of blisters under his left nipple had become infected and red lines were leading to his axillary lymph nodes which were swollen and painful. I treated him with a combination of antibacterial and antiviral antibiotics and invited him to participate in my research.

Background

Scott is slim, of average height, and looks younger than his age. During the interview he spoke hesitantly with a fixed, smiling expression and seemed to be very uncomfortable with personal questions. He is an only child whose father died of a heart attack when he was one year old, and he has never been separated from his mother who never remarried. Their relationship is good but he avoids confiding in her because she always wants to know more than he is prepared to tell her. She is very nosy. However, he feels free to come and go as he pleases and finds living with her very convenient. His confidant is a man whom he talks to on the phone once a month and whom he sees once a year.

Ongoing Stress

Three months before the eruption of his shingles one of the three technical support workers found a better-paid job and left. Since then Scott has to deal with an increased number of phone calls from customers who ring for advice, and this is not the type of work that he enjoys. He finds it annoying having to repeat the same thing again and again for people who do not understand his advice. It also seems to him that an increasing number of customers ring to complain angrily that they have been wrongly billed. His job is to work out how much must be refunded to them before he passes them on to the accounts department. He has noticed that although his colleagues can tell immediately which of the customers are angry, he is rather insensitive to their anger and this unawareness helps him to stay calm. After all, he cannot shove the money down the telephone line. Although he has been promised a rise, to compensate for his hard work, nothing has materialised yet, and the company, rather than replacing the worker who left, is thinking of employing at low cost someone from the youth training scheme who is going to do most of the boring mechanical chores.

Acute Anger at Losing his files

The work that Scott enjoys most is system administration programming. Recently he had been working on a programme that would automatically e-mail customers who were behind with their payments, and this would relieve his workload. He had been working under a lot of pressure because he had to finish it before his approaching holiday and he was taking work home every day. *Nine days before the eruption of his shingles* he was using a programme which, unbeknown to him, was corrupted by a virus, and when he tried to save his completed files the programme crashed and he lost all his files. He felt very annoyed. He experienced his annoyance as an awareness of his tongue inside his mouth and his brain inside his skull. He pursed his lips, inhaled sharply and his muscles tensed. When he realised that he could not retrieve his files he started all over again. It took him most of the week to rewrite the files he had lost, working late into the night and over the weekend. *Two days before the eruption of shingles* he managed to complete the work.

Pauline

Pauline is a nineteen-year-old, first-year university student. She is petite, with a round face and large, intelligent eyes. Her hair is drawn back in a bun and she talks in an animated, lively way.

Shingles

One day she developed a small cluster of blisters surrounded by a red patch on the skin of the left loin. Six days later the blisters spread to occupy the whole T10 dermatome, extending from the spine round the left loin and all the way to her navel. The main sensation was itching and pain was minimal.

Background

When Pauline was three years old, her eighteen-months-older sister developed a malignant cancer and died after a short illness. Pauline remembers almost nothing of the drama that surrounded these tragic events, except that she went to live with her grandparents during her sister's illness.

She became very close to them and spent most of her childhood with them until she was eleven years old, and continued to visit them for two hours every day after school. When she was twelve years old she was involved in a road traffic accident, and although she had only sustained a whiplash injury of her neck, she subsequently developed epileptic fits which, despite anti-epileptic medication, still occur at the rate of one every ten weeks.

Two years before the eruption of shingles her grandfather developed cancer of the bowel and she became very upset when she was told. She cried a lot and could not bring herself to visit him in hospital because she did not like seeing people when they are ill. She was closer to him than her grandmother, and when he died she cried inconsolably for a long time.

Ongoing Stress

Three months before the eruption of shingles her grandmother had a sudden heart attack. This time she found the courage to visit her in hospital with her mother, but it was quite a shock and she had an eerie feeling. Her stomach was turning upside down and she almost cried. For the whole week that her grandmother was in hospital she was afraid that she might die, and she did not want another grandparent to die.

Two months before the eruption of shingles, for the first time since the fits began, she has had more fits than usual, which to her is an indication of stress.

One month before the eruption of shingles her grandmother's sister died unexpectedly, but she had coped with her death much better than with the earlier heart attack.

Six months before the eruption of shingles Pauline got her A levels and was offered a place at university studying chemistry. Although she was very sad to separate from her school boyfriend who went to university in another city, she made new friends and met David, a fellow student, who became her confidant and lover, and with whom she has a very relaxing chatty relationship. He has become a major part of her life.

Acute Fear of Losing David

Life at university is quite busy, and Pauline divides her time between her parents' home and the university hall of residence. She has to study hard and prepare for two practicals a week, two lectures every day and meetings with her tutor every two weeks. Unfortunately David is lazy. He does not like getting out of bed in the morning. She has tried kicking him out of bed and dragging him to lectures, but most of the time she fails. Very often she stays with him and they ask a friend to sign them in for the lecture. David does not get on with his tutor and has been missing tutorials.

One week before the eruption of shingles David received a letter from the head of chemistry inviting him to see the Dean to discuss whether he had a future at the university. He read the letter in front of her and became quiet. She said that it was not a very nice feeling. At the time they did not know whether he was going to be thrown out of university. If he was expelled he would have to go back to his parents in the north of England and she would lose him. He is her best friend and only lover and it would be quite a loss.

Shirley

Shirley is a forty-one-year-old graphic designer who is in the process of changing career to become an actress. She is slim and attractive, wears fashionable clothes, looks younger than her age and speaks with a sexy voice.

Shingles

One day she began feeling ill, developed pain in her right loin and thought that she was developing a kidney infection. Three days later she developed a few blisters in her loin, and within the next four days the blisters spread to occupy the whole L1 dermatome from her loin to her groin.

Background

Shirley is the eldest of three children. She is seven years older than her younger sibling. Her father had a lot of financial worries and he was always short-tempered and intolerant of noise. When Shirley became a teenager she felt that she was turned into a little mother so that her mother could go to work. She had to stay in, prepare meals and clean the house. Although she tried to please her, she felt that her mother did not know how to show affection and was not protective enough of her needs. When she developed anorexia at the age of fourteen her parents did not show much concern for her health and did not take her to the doctor. She feels a resentful love for her mother, and when she talks about her parents she becomes emotional because it makes her feel neglected.

Her father died of a heart attack at the age of fifty-six when Shirley was twenty-six years old; her mother, who blamed his death on her own infidelities, started drinking excessively. She died of carcinoma of the oesophagus six years later, at the age of fifty-nine.

Shirley feels that there is a cold side to her, as there was a cold side to her mother, and she is very scared of being involved in relationships. She separated from her husband six years before the eruption of shingles and he moved out of their house leaving her alone with six cats. They remain good friends and she continues to do some work for his company occasionally.

Ongoing Stress

Three months before the eruption of shingles she went across the road to visit a neighbour for twenty minutes and when she came back her TV, her video and her stereo system had been stolen. Although she suspected her next-door neighbours of the burglary because many suspicious types had been going in and out of their house, she had no proof. For a long time she lived in fear and loathing, planning a revenge that would annihilate her neighbours so that they would not be able to retaliate. She felt so insecure in her house that she did not want to live there any more and she put the house on the market. There had always been a problem with the house next door. When she first moved into the house with her husband seven students lived in it and made an unbelievable noise. They were evicted and the house remained empty for a year and it was bliss. Then an Indian family with seven children moved in and they made a lot of noise, and now this. The house seems cursed.

Acute Fear of Feeling Unprotected

She reported the burglary to the police and she was contacted by a policeman who was friendly and chatty, and who appeared to take her suspicions seriously. This made her feel very relieved that she was not simply being paranoid. However, very soon it became clear that he was more interested in an affair with her than finding out who the burglars were. Although she found him repulsive she hesitated for a few weeks before telling him that she did not want to go out with him, because she was worried that by rejecting him she might compromise the investigation of her case. *Two weeks before the eruption of shingles*, however, she told him in no uncertain terms that she was not interested in him sexually and he passed her case on to someone else. She felt guilty for rejecting him and tainted by having led him on for so long.

Four days before the eruption of shingles another policeman came to see her and pointed out that he could not arrest or even caution her neighbours on her suspicions only. They would only deny her accusation and then she would have to continue living next to them and they might not be very friendly. At this point Shirley's heart sank and she felt vulnerable. Up until then she felt that the police were on her side because they were convinced that her neighbours had been responsible for the burglary and could at least tell them that they were under suspicion. Suddenly she felt that people could walk into her house and take things and go unpunished. She felt unprotected.

Lewis

Lewis is a forty-nine-year-old contract manager for a security firm. He is of average build, speaks with a worried expression and looks tired.

Shingles

One day Lewis felt a twinge in his left shoulder radiating down the left arm. Alarmed, he went to casualty, thinking that he was having a heart attack. However, all the tests were normal and in the next few days small blisters appeared on his shoulder and the rash spread to involve the whole of the C6 dermatome.

Background

Lewis was born in Ireland. He is the middle of three children. He married young and had two sons and a daughter, but his wife never forgave him for an affair he had had while she was grieving for the death of her father. She left him four months after the death of his mother when Lewis was thirty years old. He could not bear to see how upset his children were about their separation and, despite the beginning of a promising career in advertising, he decided to make a clean break, move to London and start his life all over again. He has not been in contact with his family since and he regrets the separation from his children who are now in their early twenties.

He lives with his second wife Jane, a secretary, who is eight years younger than he.

Three months before the eruption of shingles they exchanged contracts on a house they liked and were in the process of packing their belongings in order to move.

Unfortunately Lewis was too busy at work to help Jane with the move.

Ongoing Stress

Ten years ago Lewis started working as a security guard, and because of his easy going character he was gradually asked to take more and more responsibility until eventually he got the job of security contract manager for several prestigious buildings. He is proud of his management status and his ability to manage 300 contracts at any one time. With his hard work he has contributed to making the company successful and he has received commendations. However, he is worried about the company's ethos which does not recognise the need for enough security guards to cover all the sites. The position of the general manager is that if you need five men, hire two. The pressure to find enough staff to cover all the sites is magnified by the demand of certain customers for white security guards only, which means that to put the right person on duty he has to move several staff around. Occasionally he has had to lie and place a black guard at a site where he is not wanted, hoping that the customer will not notice.

The chronic understaffing problem demands that at times he has to ask his staff to miss their lunch break. He feels that this amounts to abuse of the people who work for the company, and although some staff accept it, others protest and walk off, leaving the place unmanned. Then Lewis has to cover the site himself. He feels unsupported by the general manager who does not care whether Lewis can cover their lunch hour, and who can take time off whenever he wants to. His attitude is that if a security guard does not like the job, someone else can be found who does. When I pointed out to Lewis that perhaps he is among those who are mistreated by the general manager he said that he is not concerned about himself. He has ways of fighting and getting round it, such as kicking a wall! Many a time he has gone into a toilet and literally kicked the wall in frustration. He has had arguments with the general manager who is putting the contract at risk. He tells Lewis that it is not his problem but Lewis believes that it is, because the men who are working for them deserve their lunch hour.

Six months before the eruption of shingles he started sweating excessively and sleeping poorly because he is constantly worrying that he may not have enough workers to cover all the sites. Although he does not feel frightened he deduces from the sweating of his armpits that he is under stress. He sweats excessively when he goes to the office first thing in the morning, and as the morning progresses and it all falls into place the sweat dries up. He does not sweat at home.

Although he is contracted to work sixty hours a week, *three months before the eruption of shingles*, two of the five contract managers left and were not replaced, so that the remaining three had to do the work of five. He started working seventy hours a week and doing night duty every third week. When he goes home at night he is exhausted. All he wants to do is sit in front of the TV.

Acute Anger at Being Let Down by the Manager

Lewis had worked seventeen hours every day for fourteen days without a break, and was looking forward to two days off which were to be covered by the general manager. *One day before the eruption of shingles*, however, the general manager rendered him speechless by telling him that because he wanted to go to a cricket match, Lewis would have to work on his days off. He growled, making a strangling gesture with his hands. 'The boss has done it again.' This was the third time that the general manager had cancelled Lewis's time off in the last three months. He says that the general manager is a version of God and there is no point arguing with God unless you want a confrontation. If he wanted this he would stand up and say: 'Bugger you, I am taking my time off.' But he is not the type of person to have a confrontation. If the general manager wants somebody to be in the office, then he'd rather be in the office than stay at home. He does not mind. He feels that somehow it is his fault that he is so easily put upon. Although he did not consider himself to be a 'yes' man, talking to me he realises that this is actually what he is.

Don

Don is a twenty-eight-year-old courier who is short, strong and stout, has a closely cropped head and talks with a thick cockney accent. He was very defensive throughout our interview because he was not used to talking about himself to anyone.

Shingles

Don had stopped having asthmatic attacks since he gave up smoking two years ago and was enjoying good health, until one day he experienced back pain and at the same time a sensation of wearing a very tight belt that was digging into his skin. Five days later, when he came to the surgery to have his pain checked out, I found an extensive blistery rash extending from his spine round the left loin, all the way to his umbilicus, the territory of the T12 dermatome.

Background

Don's parents separated when he was twelve years old and one year later his father died suddenly of a heart attack. His mother had a nervous breakdown and was admitted to hospital, and since then she relapses every two or three years. Don had been living at home with his mother and his twenty-three-year-old sister until his girlfriend Jan became pregnant three years ago, when Jan's mother invited them both to live with her.

Ongoing Stress

Jan's panic attacks disappeared while she was pregnant but returned after the birth of their daughter eighteen months ago. Don worries about her health and when she has a panic attack nearly once a week he feels helpless and stays with her until she feels better. Although Don has been a courier for the local council for eleven years his pay has not been sufficient to allow him to save or go on holidays. Therefore he decided to do an extra job, and *five months before the eruption of shingles* he started minicabbing at night. He would return home from work at 5 p.m., and would go out again at 6 p.m. and work until 1 a.m. He would return home, unwind for an hour and sleep for five hours until 7 a.m. when he had to go to work again.

Two months before the eruption of shingles his mother relapsed and was admitted to hospital. When he went to visit her he was shocked to see how drowsy the drugs she was taking had made her.

His Acute Fear of Becoming an Accomplice of a Drug Dealer

Minicabbing was stressful not only because it was depriving him of his sleep but also because occasionally some of his customers would not pay their fare and then he would feel gutted. *Three days before the eruption of shingles*, he was hired by a suspicious-looking customer who wanted to go to a rough part of London. When they arrived at their destination he got out of the car and asked Don to put the locks on the doors and wait for him until he returned. Don suspected that he was probably a drug dealer who went to collect drugs, and he felt butterflies in his stomach. He was afraid that if the police stopped him and found the drugs, they might think that he was an accomplice.

Cathy

Cathy is a thirty-five-year-old teacher of average build who has a worried expression.

Herpes Simplex? Shingles?

One day Cathy developed a small cluster of blisters the size of a 50p coin on the back of her chest at the level of T10. The pain was minimal and she complained only of itching. She had had a similar eruption in the past.

Background

Cathy is an only child whose father died of a heart attack when she was six years old. Her mother remarried, but her stepfather was a violent man and the marriage did not last long. Cathy is living with Thomas, her nine-year-old son from her first marriage, her second husband John, and their two children, two-year-old Tim and four-month-old Anna.

Ongoing stress

One year before the eruption of herpes, Cathy began feeling unwell. She was tired, felt sick and developed a pain on her left side. When the doctor eventually diagnosed pregnancy she was shocked. After three terminations she thought she was being very careful with her contraception. She decided to keep the baby, but at sixteen weeks of pregnancy when she was told that the screening test for spina bifida was positive she cried uncontrollably. Until the results of the amniocentesis and the detailed scan were known she tried to forget she was pregnant. She could not take the risk of relating to the new baby in case she needed to have an abortion. She felt that she could not give her children the attention and love they needed if all her energy was taken up by a handicapped child. Fortunately the results were normal and *four months before the eruption of herpes* she gave birth to Anna.

Two months before the eruption of herpes, Anna became unwell, went off her food and started vomiting. Cathy rushed her to Casualty and by the time the doctor examined her she was floppy and lethargic and had difficulty breathing. The doctors were very concerned, and Cathy – who by then was very frightened and in tears – thought that her baby was going to die. Anna was admitted to the intensive care unit with a diagnosis of bronchiolitis, and meningitis was eventually ruled out. *Six weeks before the eruption of Cathy's herpes*, Anna was discharged, but one day later she relapsed and had to be readmitted for another week. Cathy felt that she was being punished for the terminations she had had in the past and was rather angry with the hospital doctors for discharging Anna prematurely.

Thomas, her eldest son, who had been very jealous about all the attention his little sister was receiving, blamed himself when Anna became ill because a few days before her admission to hospital he had gone to a party where he had come into contact with a child who later developed meningitis. *Five weeks before the eruption of herpes* Cathy had an urgent call from his school informing her that Thomas had fallen in the playground and had broken his tibia.

Acute Fear of the Retrieval of an Old Memory

Two days before the eruption of herpes, Cathy had a phone call from Lina, her confidante. 'Guess who had the police here at half past two in the morning?', she said. Cathy was shocked to hear her story. She had always considered Lina's husband to be a quiet and peaceful man, but the previous night he had found a telephone number he did not recognise in the telephone's memory and suspected that his wife was having an affair. That night he woke her up at 2 a.m., told her to come with him to the kitchen, and there he pushed her against the wall and threatened to slit her throat with a kitchen knife. Fortunately Lina's little daughter heard the noise and came downstairs. When she saw what was going on she started screaming, and he switched off and walked away. After this experience Lina called the police, and because she could not trust her husband any more, she went to live with her parents in another part of London, so that they could no longer meet daily when they were taking their children to school.

Hearing about this episode stirred up Cathy's memories of her stepfather's cruelty and she became quiet and withdrawn for some time afterwards. Her stepfather was jealous of the attention his wife used to give to Cathy, and when she went out to work he would lock Cathy in her bedroom, show her a knife and tell her that if she tried to get out of the bedroom he was going to cut her up into little pieces. One day when she was eleven she was reading comics in bed and, because the ink had rubbed on to her fingers, he dragged her out of bed and beat her so hard that she ran to a friend's house for shelter and was afraid to go back home. Her friend's mother called the police who told her mother to take out an injunction against this man so that he was not allowed near Cathy again. This frightening experience made her decide never to hit her children, and even watching violence against women and children on TV gives her flashbacks.

Winnie

Winnie is a forty-seven-year-old Jamaican woman who was unemployed at the time of the interview. She looked much younger than her age.

Herpes SImplex? Shingles?

One day Winnie presented with an elongated cluster of blisters on her back, which was more itchy than painful and extended 10 cm, from the tip of her shoulder blade across dermatomes T1 and T2.

Background

Winnie is the elder of two children. She was born in Jamaica. When she was eight years old her parents emigrated to England and she was left in the care of her paternal aunt. She was very sad at separating from her mother and was afraid that she might not see her again. She did not get on well with her carers, who thought that she was a strange child and, at the age of sixteen her parents asked her to come to England to join them. Her mother was an ambitious woman who was always very busy working as a hairdresser and she did not point her in the right direction. Instead of pursuing her education and going to university, she married early and had three children.

Her mother died of kidney failure at the age of forty-four, sixteen years after they were reunited, and her father died ten years later at the age of sixty-six.

One year after her mother's death, Winnie divorced her violent husband and went to work in order to support her children. Eight years before the eruption of herpes, around the time her children were leaving home, she went through a very stressful period. She developed asthma and hypertension. Although she has a boyfriend, she prefers to live on her own. She does not discuss her problems with anyone but always tries to solve them herself.

Ongoing Stress

Winnie is tired of always scraping the bottom of the barrel and struggling to pay the bills. The £45 a week in income support she receives is just enough to buy crisps for her grandchildren. She would like to earn enough money to buy nice clothes and to save enough money to enable her to go back to her own country as soon as possible and enjoy life.

Hoping to improve her chances of finding a good job she went to college for three years, and *one year before the eruption of herpes* she earned a BTech diploma in business and finance with distinction. Her tutor urged her to go to university, but she felt that qualifying at the age of fifty-one would not improve her job prospects.

However, despite her qualifications she has not had much luck with job applications. She has experienced a lot of prejudice in her life, but recently she has become very conscious of her age. She has been to many interviews but the jobs are given to younger people who do not have her qualifications, and she finds this humiliating and unfair. She feels very angry when she is treated in this way. When she was younger she used to lose her temper and get into a lot of arguments and fights. But gradually she has learnt to contain her anger and keep it inside her, but she has asthma attacks instead.

Eight months before the eruption of herpes her daughter told her that she was pregnant again and Winnie was very disappointed that she had decided to have another baby so soon after the first one. She had wanted her to further her education and get on with her career. She helped her with the first baby, but she was not prepared to do so with the second because she herself wanted to find a job and earn some money.

Six months before the eruption of herpes she came home one day and found the door of her flat kicked in. Burglars had searched the flat but had not stolen anything. She became angry, shouting at anybody and everybody, and told the police that they had better book a cell for her in Holloway prison because if she caught the burglars she would kill them. She calmed down after a few days, and *five months before the eruption of herpes* she found a job as a receptionist with additional light cleaning duties at a local hospital. *Four months before the eruption of herpes*, while she was still learning the job, the senior receptionist saw her photocopying a certificate for a patient and told her off angrily in front of the other receptionists. Winnie managed to keep her anger inside and not shout back, but she told her in no uncertain terms that she did not like being made to feel stupid in front of her colleagues. When the supervisor asked her a few days later why she was so angry with the senior receptionist, Winnie replied that if she had really been angry with her, she would have had to go to India to pick her up, because that was how far she would have kicked her. She demanded to be treated with respect or else they would see the other side of her, which is not very nice. She told the supervisor that the job was not so important to her that she would have to put up with humiliating behaviour. She had qualifications and she could find a job elsewhere. After this episode she became progressively dissatisfied with her job because the supervisor was putting pressure on her to do more and more cleaning work for the same salary.

Acute Anger and Fear at the Second Workplace

Three weeks before the eruption of herpes, she took a cleaning job for two hours every morning starting at 5.30 a.m., on top of her job as a receptionist. However, very soon she felt unfairly treated because the supervisor gave her more work to do than the two cleaners who had already been working there and who wasted a lot of time laughing and joking with each other. *One week before the eruption of herpes* she complained to the manager, who saw her point and tried to divide the work equally between all three of them. However, one of the cleaners started shouting and being grumpy and soon went on sick leave with back pain. Winnie had to cover the duties of the absent worker and face the supervisor and the other cleaner who were both hostile to her. She felt resentful, and when she told the supervisor that her doctor had diagnosed an infection with the chickenpox virus, the supervisor told her to take sick leave and stay away from her because she had a young baby at home.

CONCLUSION

If alexithymia and depression seem unlikely to be risk factors for the eruption of herpes zoster, what is the emotional context within which shingles erupts? The stories above illustrate that shingles does not erupt out of the blue, but is preceded by a number of stressful events and difficulties which produce a baseline of negative emotions that magnify each other and lead to an emotional experience of toxic intensity. In this emotional climate any experience of a new intense negative emotion can push a person beyond the limits of tolerance. Nathanson has pointed out that when, in the context of a social or interpersonal situation, emotion is piled on emotion, one magnifying the other continuously, the resulting intensity of emotion can be unbearable and the individual may become inconsolable. Just as the heat of a nuclear fusion engine bears little relationship to the flames in our fireplace that heat us in winter, emotion at its highest magnification does not resemble the basic innate emotions but represents a disregulation of affect which in turn can disregulate other bodily systems, including the immune system. Although none of the patients I have seen so far have developed post-herpetic neuralgia, it would be foolish to claim that my psychosomatic attitude protected them. To research such a possibility would involve the study of a greater number of shingles patients than a general practitioner can see in a lifetime. But my findings so far suggest that shingles follows the kind of life disruption that could also precede other potentially serious infections such as pneumonia. Armed with the above knowledge we can offer patients who develop shingles more help than an accurate diagnosis and antiviral medication of doubtful efficacy (Lancaster et al. 1995). We can ask them whether they have experienced any previous losses or been under stress recently and then listen to their stories with interest, sympathy and understanding. This medical activity can provide solace and induce calm, as Michael and Enid Balint have repeatedly demonstrated. Thomas, the first of the shingles patients presented here, told me later that he experienced the research interview as an important therapeutic intervention. Brody has argued in a very interesting paper that the general practitioner has the power to implement symbolic healing by listening carefully to a patient's story and engaging with the patient in the joint task of construction of narrative (Brody 1994). The doctor who listens carefully to the patient's story of suffering lays the groundwork for the important dimensions of symbolic healing. These include an explanatory system, care and compassion, and mastery and control. Giving the patient an accurate explanation of his disease or illness allows him to participate more actively in his treatment; demonstrating care and compassion may give the patient the reassurance that he needs to participate in this way; and finally, instilling a sense of power and control is vital if the patient is to feel truly empowered and able to take specific actions that will promote health and ameliorate symptoms. The joint construction of narrative may also contribute to cognitive processing of traumatic emotional memories stored in non-declarative memory so that they can be stored in declarative or narrative memory, retrieval from which is not accompanied by the strong physical manifestations of traumatic emotions.

5 BREATHING AND FEELING: ADAPTIVE HANDLING OF HYPERVENTILATION SYNDROME IN GENERAL PRACTICE

> The soul breathes through the body and suffering, whether it starts in the skin or in a mental image, happens in the flesh.
>
> Antonio Damasio, *Descartes' Error.*

ANXIETY OR HYPERVENTILATION SYNDROME: THE CHICKEN OR THE EGG?

One of the challenges I faced when I started working in general practice was to develop a constructive approach to patients who presented with anxiety about a multitude of physical symptoms which did not fit the pattern of a recognisable medical disease. Their symptoms seemed real enough and most of the time suggested serious respiratory or cardiac disease, but clinical examination and laboratory investigations did not support such a diagnosis. Just telling the patients that there was nothing wrong with their lungs or heart made them feel that the doctor probably thought that they were imagining their symptoms or that they were going mad. Learning about hyperventilation syndrome, however, provided me not only with a way of making sense of my patients' symptoms but also with a method of helping patients control them.

Hyperventilation syndrome is one of the commonest causes of functional symptoms. There is also the suggestion that it may cause coronary vasospasm leading to cardiac arrhythmias and myocardial infarction in patients with ischaemic heart disease (Weiner 1991).

Hospital-based researchers claim that it is the cause of attendance of 6–10 per cent of patients in medical outpatient clinics (Lum 1976). Although Burton (1993) had found that hyperventilation-induced symptoms were common in a group of twenty patients presenting to their general practitioner with recurrent functional symptoms which doctors had found difficult to treat, nobody knew what its prevalence was in general practice. In 1992 I decided to record all patients diagnosed and treated with this syndrome over a year. There were 100 such patients, the observations on whom are reported in this chapter. Since then I have found that about 4–6 per cent of my consultations each year are taken up with the management of patients suffering from the syndrome.

WHAT IS HYPERVENTILATION SYNDROME?

The term 'ventilation' refers to the function that satisfies the body's need for oxygen. The term 'hyperventilation' means ventilation in excess of the body's need for oxygen. The term 'hyperventilation syndrome', however, has nothing to do with oxygen. It refers to the multitude of symptoms which are produced when irregular, sighing, upper thoracic breathing of which the patient is unaware causes carbon dioxide deficiency. Persistently lowered and fluctuating levels of carbon dioxide in the blood are critical as they are responsible for most of the symptoms of which the patient complains (Lum 1987). The key factor for the initiation of the syndrome is the type of breathing. Upper thoracic breathing is part of the somatic component of emotional arousal. It occurs when prolonged, intense, affective states of which the patient is unaware, such as panic, rage and sorrow, cannot be expressed in automatic action, such as running to escape, fighting to kill or howling in anguish. These powerful emotions threaten to overwhelm the patient and create a sense of helplessness. Once the hyperventilation syndrome is initiated it can be sustained by several factors other than the original emotional arousal and a vicious circle may set in. Among these factors are secondary anxiety about the significance of the symptoms and the doctor's inability to make the correct diagnosis. John Bowlby has given us a fascinating account of the life of Charles Darwin, whose hyperventilation symptoms baffled his physicians. Their inability to explain them and treat them became a risk factor for their maintenance (Bowlby 1990). Another risk factor that can contribute to the maintenance of hyperventilation syndrome is maladaptive health beliefs; for example, that upper thoracic breathing helps relaxation, or that the symptoms are due to lack of oxygen. These can make patients intensify their ventilatory efforts and make the symptoms worse. A less frequent misconception is that the symptoms are due to too much oxygen. For example, Angela Wilkie, a well informed journalist, in her book *Having Cancer and How to Live With It* (1993), observed that in her panic about a possible recurrence of ovarian cancer she began to hyperventilate, but she attributed her lightheadedness wrongly to getting too much oxygen into her system.

Habitual sighing, sniffing or yawning in an attempt to relieve unpleasant upper chest tightness can also increase ventilation. There is also evidence that hyperventilation can become chronic when central control mechanisms develop which actively prevent carbon dioxide from returning to normal levels. Any increase in carbon dioxide due to reduction of ventilation is then opposed by a drive to increase ventilation mediated by the chemoreceptors in the body which detect carbon dioxide levels in the blood.

SYMPTOMS OF HYPERVENTILATION SYNDROME

Here I summarise most of the known clinical manifestations of hyperventilation syndrome in order of frequency of presentation in the 100 consecutive hyperventilating patients whom I treated in 1992 (Zalidis 1994a).

Respiratory

- Sensation of breathlessness which occurs typically at rest or after, but not during exertion.
- Inability to take a deep enough breath.
- Chest tightness.
- Dry, irritable cough with frequent clearing of the throat.
- Excessive sighing, frequent yawning.
- Frequent sniffing.
- Excessive use of upper chest and accessory muscles of respiration.
- Waking up around 3 o'clock in the morning and fighting for breath.

Neurological

- Light-headedness and dizziness.
- Sensations of numbness and/or tingling anywhere, but especially at fingertips, toes and around the mouth.
- Blurred vision.
- Sudden loss of consciousness.
- Headaches.
- Intolerance of bright lights and loud noise.

Cardiovascular

- Palpitations, missed heartbeats, racing heart.
- Dull upper-right or upper-left chest pains.
- Areas of thoracic tenderness.
- Fainting due to postural hypotension.

General

- Feeling tired all the time, weakness.
- Poor concentration, forgetfulness.
- Poor sleep, nightmares.
- Excessive sweating, particularly in armpits and palms.
- Cold extremities.
- Warm feelings in the head.

Musculoskeletal

- Aching all over.
- Increased muscle tone with muscle stiffness.
- Cramps.
- Tremors or coarse twitching, shivering.
- Occasionally carpal and pedal spasms.
- Rarely, generalised and involuntary painful muscular spasms, also known as tetany.

Gastrointestinal

- Frequent swallowing leading to aerophagy.
- Dry mouth.

- Difficulty in swallowing.
- Sensation of lump in the throat.
- Full or bloated abdominal sensations.
- Belching.
- Heartburn due to oesophageal reflux.
- Sharp lower chest pains, accentuated by breathing.

Psychological

- Tension.
- Anxiety.
- Depersonalisation.
- Panic attacks.
- Phobic states.
- Fear of insanity.

CAUSES OF HYPERVENTILATION SYNDROME

Pfeffer has categorised the causes of hyperventilation into four groups: organic, physiological, habit and emotional (Pfeffer 1978). Organic causes include drug effects, early stages of alcohol withdrawal and central nervous system lesions. Physiological causes include altitude acclimatisation, heat and exercise. In general practice, however, hyperventilation is most commonly associated with emotional arousal, which was identified in eighty-four of my patients; only two were hyperventilating as a result of taking drugs such as ecstasy or cocaine.

AGE AND SEX DISTRIBUTION

Of my patients, sixty-nine were women and thirty-one were men; twenty-three were in their twenties, thirty-two were in their thirties and eighteen in their forties. The numbers were much lower for those aged ten or less and for those aged fifty and over. The youngest hyperventilating patient I saw was four years old and the eldest was eighty-three.

Of the ninety who came to the surgery, forty presented as emergencies without having made a previous appointment; ten patients felt so incapacitated and frightened by their symptoms that they asked for a home visit.

HOW DO HYPERVENTILATING PATIENTS PRESENT?

Forty-one patients presented with respiratory symptoms, particularly chest tightness, or an inability to take a deep enough breath. Most patients had some difficulty in describing these sensations and used a variety of images in their effort to convey their meaning.

Some complained of a tight elastic band around their chest, or a heavy weight preventing the chest from expanding, or of thick tenacious mucous preventing it from expanding from inside. Others complained of a sensation of blockage which stopped the air from going into their chest which they sometimes attempted to dislodge by coughing or putting their fingers in their throat to make themselves sick. Occasionally patients used the words 'chest pains' to describe chest tightness, and without a detailed description of their symptoms they might have been misdiagnosed. Very often patients thought that they had a chest infection or asthma and demanded antibiotics. Another common complaint was that they were suffering from lack of oxygen.

There were twenty-seven patients who presented with neurological symptoms, particularly light-headedness, numbness and tingling. Pins and needles or tingling does not have to be symmetrical or bilateral and can occur in any part of the body. When the pins and needles affect the upper arms, they can be confused with the pain of myocardial ischaemia. Chest pains occurred in fourteen patients, and twelve patients complained of feeling tired all the time and aching all over. These symptoms suggested a flu-like illness, and some patients wondered whether they suffered from ME (myalgic encephalomyelitis). Two patients presented with gastrointestinal symptoms such as the sensation of a lump in the throat or abdominal bloating. Only one patient presented with painful, generalised, involuntary muscle spasms, a condition known in medical terms as tetany that is the result of extreme hyperventilation.

DIAGNOSIS

I agree with Magarian (1982), Lum (1987) and Paulley (1990) that hyper-ventilation syndrome is a clinical diagnosis. When a patient anxiously complains of frightening physical symptoms such as chest pain or breathing difficulty, the non-verbal communication is one of fear. In order to proceed with the consultation in a constructive way, I have to tolerate my own fear that I may be in the presence of a medical catastrophe, as well as the patient's fear that is communicated through his body language. I have to critically examine the urge to take immediate action to rule out such a possibility, tolerating the fear long enough for the patient to describe his presenting symptoms in as much detail as possible. I also ask him to say what he is afraid may be wrong with him in order to help him to verbalise his emotions.

When I suspect from the way the patient is describing the symptoms that he may be suffering from hyperventilation syndrome, I ask whether there are any other symptoms. Patients usually focus on a few symptoms only – they do not volunteer them all; either because they do not consider them relevant or because they are afraid that the doctor may make an unfavourable diagnosis. For this reason, when I suspect the diagnosis I find it essential to ask in an orderly and systematic way for all the symptoms of hyperventilation syndrome, taking one organ system at a time, and paying attention not only to what the patient says but also to how he says it, to his body language. I am alert to the clues that are suggestive of hyperventilation syndrome, such as frequent sniffing, sighing, dry cough, yawning or constant clearing of the throat. The finding of characteristic multiple symptoms is the most useful aid in the diagnosis of hyperventilation syndrome. In fact the greater the number of corroborative symptoms, the more likely it is that this is the diagnosis.

Only after having exhausted the symptom list do I examine the patient. I listen to the heart and lungs, check the blood pressure and record the peak expiratory flow rate (PEFR) where this seems relevant. Then I ask the patient to lie down on the couch to observe the respiratory pattern. Upper thoracic breathing is another corroborative sign. In chronic hyperventilators a urine test may show a strong alkaline reaction reflecting the excretion of sodium bicarbonate which compensates for the loss of carbon dioxide.

A careful history and a physical examination are essential aspects of the management because they give the patient confidence that his fears of organic disease have been taken into account. They are also essential if the doctor is not to miss one of the diagnoses that hyperventilation syndrome can superficially mimic. For example, a fifty-year old woman came to the surgery because she thought she had had a chest infection for four weeks and it was not getting better. When I asked her to describe her symptoms, she told me that she kept getting stabbing chest pains when walking, together with a sense of a weight or tightness in her chest. She also felt that she could not take a deep enough breath. This is the typical way in which hyperventilation syndrome sufferers complain of their sense of breathlessness. She was also breathless on exertion. On systematic questioning, however, the only other symptom I could elicit was tiredness. On auscultation, she had diminished breath sounds on the right side of the chest, with normal resonance on percussion. My clinical diagnosis was pneumothorax, or in other words, collapsed lung. A chest X-ray confirmed the diagnosis and her management was taken over by the chest physicians.

The explanation of hyperventilation is so different from what the patient expects to hear that some patients will need to be convinced. This is best done by asking the patient to make himself carbon dioxide deficient in the presence of the doctor by taking fast and deep breaths for about three minutes. Most patients give up after less than one minute, because this manoeuvre reproduces their very unpleasant symptoms in a most convincing manner. A word of caution: voluntary hyperventilation is to be avoided in patients with known or suspected ischaemic heart disease because of the risk of inducing coronary vasospasm which may lead to arrhythmias and even myocardial infarction.

PATHOPHYSIOLOGY

I find that understanding the physiology of hyperventilation symptoms helps me to appreciate their somatic nature. I have therefore summarised some of the pathophysiological mechanisms from several major papers (Lum 1976, Evans and Lum 1981, Magarian 1982, Freeman and Nixon 1985, Nixon 1994).

One of the most common presenting symptoms, air hunger, or the sense of being unable to take a deep enough breath, is due to the characteristic over-inflation of the chest. Attempting to inflate the lungs from a position above the resting one is opposed by the elastic forces of the rib cage and demands extra effort which is interpreted as inspiratory difficulty, evoking the desire for even larger breaths. Overfilling of the upper chest can cause compression of the subclavian artery between the first rib and the clavicle leading to ischaemic pain that affects the whole arm and hand, and may also cause paresthesiae and sensory impairment affecting all the fingers.

Carbon dioxide deficiency and respiratory alkalosis develop rapidly after the onset of hyperventilation. Carbon dioxide, far from being a waste gas, plays a very important role in regulating vital body systems. It is a major factor in governing cerebral blood flow. Cerebral angiography has demonstrated that arterial and venous vasoconstriction, causing a reduction of the cerebral blood flow, is the initial response to hyperventilation, leading to cerebral anoxia. The hypoxia is made worse by tighter binding of oxygen to the haemoglobin in the presence of alkalosis so that it is not easily available to the tissues. The resulting symptoms are dizziness, light-headedness, disturbance of consciousness, syncope, hallucinations, and visual phenomena such as blurred vision, tunnel vision, flashing lights or even complete blackout. In time the initial vasoconstriction is overcome by the cerebrovascular vasodilatory response to anoxia and the symptoms disappear. If low levels of carbon dioxide and respiratory alkalosis are sustained, renal compensation occurs through increased renal excretion of bicarbonate in order to maintain the pH of the blood at its normal value of 7.4. When severe, the depletion of the alkaline reserves in the muscles causes fatigue and loss of the capacity for physical effort through the diminution of the buffering effect on lactic acid. Common symptoms are fatigue and aching limbs. The unbuffered acid is carried centrally and stimulates further over-breathing. Chronic depletion of the alkaline buffering system produced by prolonged excessive loss of carbon dioxide causes pH regulation to be sensitive to small changes in breathing. When breathing is reduced during the first hours of sleep, acidosis develops. At a critical point this reduction in pH triggers an overbreathing response and wakens the subject with hypocapnia. The consequences can include anxiety, panic, sleepwalking, nausea, muscular pains or cramps, cardiac pain or arrhythmias, or both. In highly aroused subjects there is a diuresis of magnesium ions. This loss of nature's own calcium blocker reduces opposition to the rise of intracellular calcium ionisation that is induced by the respiratory alkalosis of hyperventilation and thereby promotes vasoconstriction.

When a chronic persistent state of hyperventilation occurs there appears to be a resetting of the respiratory centre, allowing for persistence of carbon dioxide tension at hypocapnic levels to preserve a normal pH. This may be one of the factors that facilitates chronicity and the ready provocation of symptoms. If there is chronic carbon dioxide deficiency, symptoms may be present much of the time or be triggered by occasional deep breaths such as a sigh or a yawn which cause minimal reductions of the already lowered carbon dioxide tension.

Because they can hyperventilate without a visibly increased respiratory rate, hyperventilators are often unrecognised. In the presence of hyperventilation, intracellular shifts of phosphate quickly cause hypophosphataemia with resulting symptoms that can mimic numerous neurological and psychiatric disorders, such as aching all over, malaise, dizziness, paresthesiae, decreased attention span and disorientation. Intracellular shifts of carbon dioxide and calcium decrease extracellular calcium and increase the intracellular pH of the neurone. This can increase neuronal activity and lead to paresthesiae, increased muscle irritability and finally tetany. Striated muscle as well as smooth muscle can be affected. Recent studies of the effect of hyperventilation on the cardiovascular system have shown that it depends on how long it lasts. Hypocapnic alkalosis induced in a normal person by voluntary hyperventilation produces a reduction in systematic resistance and mean arterial blood pressure, with an increase in cardiac output and heart rate. These changes are maximal at one minute, minimal at four minutes and completely absent by seven minutes. As the above changes can be blocked by an antihistamine and not by a beta-blocker, it is suggested that the cardiovascular responses to hyperventilation are mediated by histamine release.

Hyperventilation can cause electrocardiographic changes such as T-wave flattening and QT prolongation as a result of respiratory alkalosis. It can also cause a more marked S-T segment depression which may be due to hypoxia. There is evidence that hypocapnic alkalosis from hyperventilation can interfere with myocardial oxygen supply, at least in patients with atherosclerotic artery disease, by producing coronary artery vasoconstriction and increasing oxygen affinity to haemoglobin.

Another feature of the electrocardiogram is the markedly increased incidence of ventricular ectopic contractions. The subjective experience of a single ectopic is uncomfortable and recurrent ectopics are commonly reported as painful.

Five causes of chest pain have been identified in patients who hyperventilate. The commonest type of pain my patients complain about is a dull aching or soreness of the right or left upper chest wall, which may radiate to the head, neck, back, shoulders or arms. When it spreads to the face or limbs it may be described as a numb feeling and may be difficult to dissociate from paresthesiae developing independently. As a rule the duration of the pain differs from that of angina. The discomfort is often present for hours at a time and sometimes days. The patient may also complain of sharp stabs, often punctuating a dull background pain. Tight constricting or burning sensations are common. The cause of this first type of pain is muscular and is due to overuse of the upper thoracic respiratory muscles, with subsequent fatigue. In addition, extracellular alkalosis increases the tendency of the skeletal muscle to develop spasms. Firm pressure at costochondral junctions or intercostal spaces locates tender areas which indicate the site of muscular spasm.

A less common cause of chest pain is mechanical from aerophagy which produces sharp, stabbing, low chest pain, which gets worse on deep breathing and results in rapid but more shallow respiration. This pain is probably caused by pressure on the diaphragm of a distended stomach or spasm of the diaphragm itself.

A third type of pain is reported in the left sub-mammary area and occurs when there is high sympathetic tone. The resultant tachycardia is perceived as heavy and uncomfortable. The forceful adrenergic slap of the heart against the chest wall may produce a tender area at the apex.

A fourth variety is due to catecholamine myopathy. Chronic high cate-cholamine levels may induce small areas of focal necrosis and scarring of the subendocardium, increasing left ventricular stiffness, reducing compliance and predisposing to pain and even infarction.

The fifth type of pain is true myocardial pain and is due to ischaemia. It can be produced in some hyperventilators by a combination of the Bohr effect and coronary vasoconctriction which decreases coronary blood flow.

Low carbon dioxide levels are also responsible for a selective depression of parasympathetic activity so that the patient presents a picture of sympathetic dominance; dilated pupils, cold hands and feet, sweating of the palms and armpits, tachycardia, passing urine frequently, and so on. With very low carbon dioxide levels these signs disappear. Some of the gastrointestinal man-ifestations of hyperventilation are due to mouth breathing and aerophagy, leading to dry mouth, sensation of lump in the throat, bloated abdominal sensations, excessive eructation and flatus and sometimes sharp, stabbing, low chest pain which gets worse on deep breathing.

BREATHING AND FEELING

Affects are always about doing something and they are expressed in action. Expressive motor behaviours associated with emotions should be thought of as action tendencies, which if actualised or fully expressed would result in overt behaviour. Whereas the activity of the muscles of facial expression is behaviour that is specific for each affect, the activity of the accessory respiratory muscles involved in upper chest breathing is non-specific and is part of the neuroendocrine and behavioural affect responses geared to whatever physiological support is required for vigorous physical action. When the patient cannot modulate the impulse to express an emotion in action, and this action is forbidden; when the patient cannot run, fight or otherwise deal with his enemies both internalised and external in any meaningful, self-saving way, he remains trapped in a chronically stressed state, in a posture of mobilisation, with all its tissue destructiveness. If he is not aware that he is in the grip of an emotion, he may become afraid that the accompanying somatic sensations indicate a medical illness. Such unawareness is more likely when non-verbalisable, primitive affect memories are retrieved, whose somatic component is very strong and which are experienced at a sensorimotor level of emotional awareness, as vague physical symptoms.

Krystal (1998) has used the term *affect regression* to describe the experience of intense, unmodulated, primitive emotions, without verbalisation or awareness of their precise nature. This notion is very close to the concept of alexithymia and indeed, Krystal considers alexithymia to be either a regressive phenomenon or an arrest of emotional development.

Another reason for experiencing the physiological element of an affect as an illness is *regression in the manner of handling affects*. The opposite attitude, *affect tolerance* – the capacity to have feelings comfortably – involves a variety of resources and actions that make possible the conscious experience of affects. People who can comfortably experience a feeling are generally secure that their emotional state is justified by their experience; that it makes sense; and that having accomplished its purpose or run its course, it will stop. People who recognise the source and meaning of their intense feelings, for example, the reaction following a near-accident or bereavement, are much less likely to engage in maladaptive handling of their affects, and the emotion runs its natural short-lived course.

People who are afraid or ashamed of their feelings, however, engage in a vicious circle of maladaptive handling of their emotions by becoming angry with themselves, or frightened, or depressed about having an affect. This attitude towards their feelings may set up a self-perpetuating circular reaction of being afraid of being afraid. This difficulty occurs more frequently with painful feelings, but some people develop a fear of all emotions, even of being in love or becoming sexually excited.

An emotion allowed to overwhelm a person at some earlier time is subsequently experienced as dangerous and is defended against. In the permanent blocking of affectivity by strong defences, the emotions are experienced as physiological 'attacks' and may break through intermittently. Even recurring periods of depression or anxiety are experienced as such 'attacks' during which the affects may not be consciously recognised as such. This subjective experience, is the cause of the tendency found in both doctors and their patients to experience their emotions as if they were illnesses. Those adults who experience affects as 'attacks' suspend their self-regulatory and self-monitoring functions, especially early in the episode.

The hyperventilation syndrome is an example of a psychosomatic condition caused by maladaptive handling of emotions. When a patient dreads that his magical powers may make the wish contained in the cognitive component of an affect come true, or being flooded by affect precursors which might overwhelm his rational behaviour and disorganise him, he experiences his affects at an undifferentiated somatic level. Irregular upper thoracic breathing is just such an undifferentiated motor expression of the impulse to express an affect in action and represents a posture of mobilisation. This kind of breathing very quickly causes symptoms due to low and fluctuating levels of carbon dioxide. The patient focuses his attention on these symptoms so that the message contained in the cognitive part of the emotion is lost. Secondary anxiety about the possible medical significance of the symptoms stimulates more upper thoracic breathing and as the self-regulating and self-monitoring functions of the individual are suspended; he becomes locked in a vicious circle.

I have learned from respiratory physiotherapists and clinical psychologists that the most effective way of breaking this vicious circle is to reverse the physiological effects of the upper chest breathing. This is best done not by asking the patient to breathe into a brown paper bag, but by encouraging him to change his breathing pattern from upper thoracic to diaphragmatic, thus changing his emotional posture from one of mobilisation, to one of tranquillity (Cluff 1984, Bradley 1992, Wilson 1999).

Kestenberg uses a similar therapy involving psychological and tactile methods during which patients are instructed to imagine that the physician's touching palm is part of their own body. She found that this technique activates diaphragmatic breathing, improves circulation and relaxes the muscles. Kestenberg emphasised that regular diaphragmatic breathing underlies the attitude of trust the infant conveys when it lies happily in its mother's lap. When an adult puts a hand on a trusting baby's belly, he feels pleasure. The tummy seems to cuddle into the softly pressing hand. The trustful attitude of stretching toward the other, of going out of one's boundaries seeking out and melting into the other person, Kestenberg has called 'transensus' (Kestenberg 1978). This physical contact between doctor and patient, during which the doctor regulates the breathing of the patient, is a form of holding, and is founded on the idea of mutual trust between mother and child (Zalidis 1992). It operates in the potential space between mother and infant where fantasy was active and love could be experienced without guilt or shame (Winnicott 1972).

Taylor (1987) has helped us understand the nature of the creative potential space between the mother's and the child's psychic reality by drawing our attention to Hofer's discoveries of hidden regulatory processes (Hofer 1983).

Hofer has shown that the early mother–infant relationship is a relatively open system in which some aspects of the infant's physiology, such as heartbeat, breathing, temperature control, growth, movement, and so on, are regulated by the mother's actions and what she provides. In turn, the baby's responses influence the behaviour of the mother.

In a similar manner, the doctor, by his behaviour, can regulate the breathing pattern of his patient and contribute to an attenuation of the patient's physiological arousal. If the doctor is interested in his patient's feelings and ideas, he can invite him, when his overwhelming physical symptoms have subsided, to come back with a longer appointment in order to talk about his emotions so that he can recognise them as a self-experience.

Because verbalisation reduces somatisation, the greater the opportunity to think and talk about feelings with a skilled therapist, the less intense the somatic response may become and the greater the opportunity to acquaint the patient with his emotions as signals to himself, often unpleasant but manageable and essentially self-limiting. Subjectively experienced emotions are the conscious awareness of synthesis of all three affect responses and they motivate adaptive behaviour rather than cause automatic reflex action.

Charlotte Balkanyi (1964) and Robert Furman (1978) are among the psychoanalysts who have emphasised the importance of expressing emotions in verbal language for distinguishing between them and for reducing and grading the intensity of their physical components.

SIX STEPS IN MANAGING HYPERVENTILATION SYNDROME

Patients who present with symptoms of hyperventilation syndrome are worried about the cause of their symptoms, are not aware of their breathing pattern and have no conscious control over it. They feel at the mercy of an alien force that has invaded their body from outside, such as a poison or a virus, or feel that they suffer from a fatal disease which is out of control.

The first step of their management is therefore to elicit all their symptoms and their fears about them.

The second step is to examine the patients. This is the most effective reassurance because patients feel that their fears about physical disease have been taken into account and considered seriously. It is also a safeguard against making the wrong diagnosis.

The third step is making the diagnosis and explaining to the patients that their symptoms are real and there is one factor that can explain them all, namely carbon dioxide deficiency, which is caused by their dysfunctional breathing pattern.

The fourth step is persuading the patients that this is indeed so. The most effective way of going about it is to ask them to make themselves carbon dioxide deficient in the presence of the doctor, by hyperventilating voluntarily for three minutes at a rate of thirty breaths per minute. This manoeuvre is also a direct way of helping patients become aware that they play an active part in the development of their symptoms.

The fifth step involves making patients aware of their upper chest breathing by pointing out the sighing respirations and teaching them to breathe with the diaphragm only.

This activity has a calming effect, which is explained partly by the fact that diaphragmatic breathing is an activator of the parasympathetic component of the autonomic system, which modulates the intensity of the sympathetic component of emotional arousal.

Whereas the first five steps of the management deal with the patients' secondary anxiety about the significance of their symptoms, the sixth step begins to address the primary anxiety which is related to the patients' panic about experiencing affects.

They panic because of the danger that they might be flooded, overwhelmed and disorganised by the affect precursors and re-experience the helplessness they felt during traumatic experiences in the past. Or they panic because they are afraid that their aggressive and sexual wishes contained in the cognitive aspect of their affects will come true – a residue of omnipotent primary process thinking.

The sixth step, therefore, involves inviting patients to engage in a relaxed conversation about their feelings in the hope that, by using language to express their emotions, they will counteract the somatisation process by mentalising them through a continuing cognitive and symbolic elaboration of their emotional arousal.

I have found that to complete the six steps of the management and deal with both the somatic and the emotional aspects of the problem needs a minimum of three sessions of at least twenty minutes each. But although this is the ideal way to manage the hyperventilation syndrome, in practice it is not always possible to do so. When I was studying hyperventilation syndrome in general practice, only fifty out of 100 attended for three or more consultations. I suspect that the reason why twenty-five patients attended only once and twenty-five twice, may be related to their basic difficulty in experiencing feelings. It is also possible that some patients are just content to be reassured that their symptoms are not due to a life-threatening disease. In the following two examples I present the initial consultations of two cases in order to illustrate my way of handling hyperventilation syndrome in the general practice setting.

TWO CLINICAL EXAMPLES

Claire

First Session: Making the Diagnosis

Claire was thirty-two years old when she came to the surgery with her daughter one day, wanting to see the doctor urgently. While they were waiting I could hear them both coughing loudly. The mother would start a coughing bout and the daughter would follow soon after. The coughing was loud and intrusive and distracted me from concentrating on the problems of the patients to be seen before them. When they finally came into the consulting room, Claire's round face and hoarse voice initially conveyed a lot of irritability. When I asked her what the problem was, she told me in an annoyed tone of voice that she had a breathing difficulty and that her asthma pumps were no good. All she wanted was different ones. As she was not responding to her asthma medication I began to doubt whether her breathing difficulty was caused by asthma, and so I asked her to describe it.

She told me between coughing bouts that her chest was tight and she was puffing away like mad trying to catch her breath. I noted the dramatic description of her symptoms and I asked her to describe her difficulty a little bit more accurately. She said that it felt as though she could not take a deep enough breath. I asked if she had any other symptoms and she volunteered that sometimes her heart was ticking away as if it was in her head. Then she was silent. Her silence was interrupted by bouts of dry, irritating coughing, and every bout triggered a similar one in her daughter. She found this very annoying because she thought that her daughter was copying her. The description of her breathlessness as well as her annoyance and the multiple symptoms made me think of the possibility of hyperventilation syndrome. I sensed her irritability and made an effort to resist its contagious nature by asking in a systematic way for the presence of characteristic symptoms from other organ systems.

I asked her whether she felt dizzy, and she admitted that she felt dizzy all the time and that this was worse when she stood up. I asked whether she had pins and needles in her fingertips, and she said that both her hands felt tingly. When I asked whether she felt tired, she admitted that she felt tired all the time. When she talked to somebody for some time she became out of breath, and when she walked or did simple things at home she felt tired. I asked whether she slept well at night and she said that she slept poorly. She tossed and turned and coughed. She woke up at 3 o'clock every morning feeling that she could not catch her breath. When I asked her if she had indigestion she said that she got heartburn and she had the feeling that there was something in her throat that stopped her from getting air into her lungs. She felt that if she poked her finger into her throat she would dislodge it. She also admitted that she was suffering from headaches and muscle cramps, that she was shaky and irritable, and that when she felt dizzy she sighed a lot, and when she felt tired she yawned a lot.

'Do these symptoms worry you?', I asked.

'Of course they worry me', she replied.

'What are you afraid may be wrong with you?'

'I am terrified that you may think I have circulation trouble', she answered.

After I elicited all these symptoms I felt more confident about the diagnosis of hyperventilation syndrome. I checked her blood pressure, recorded her PEFR and listened to her chest. Everything was normal.

I asked her to lie on the couch and observed her breathing pattern, which was predominantly upper thoracic.

I told her that I had good news for her. Her symptoms were not due to lung disease or circulation trouble, but rather to carbon dioxide deficiency which was brought on by her upper chest breathing.

She looked at me in a rather puzzled way. I went on to explain that chest breathing is emergency breathing. It is the kind of breathing we do when we want to run or fight or scream or cry. If we breathe like this without doing any of these things, then we blow out more carbon dioxide than we need to and we develop frightening symptoms.

'Do you know what carbon dioxide is?', I asked her. As she did not, I explained that oxygen is what we breathe in; carbon dioxide is what we breathe out – the exhaust fumes of the body so to speak. But unlike exhaust fumes, it is not all bad. The body needs a certain amount to function properly. If you breathe out too much, then you feel ill. The way to stop this happening is to begin breathing with your diaphragm. Normal, relaxing breathing is diaphragmatic.

I asked her if she knew what the diaphragm is and as she did not, I asked her to imagine that if her chest was a barrel, then the bottom of the barrel would be her diaphragm. Just as the heart is the circulation muscle of the body, the diaphragm is the main breathing muscle, a dome-shaped muscle that separates the lungs from the gut, that moves up and down and causes breathing.

'It is about here', I told her putting my hand on her abdomen and pressing down gently but firmly. 'To breathe with your diaphragm blow your tummy up as the air goes in though your nose and slowly push my hand up with your tummy. Try to breathe in and out slowly about six times a minute.'

She tried a few times, looking rather incredulous and bewildered.

This look on the patient's face usually prompts me to demonstrate the effects of carbon dioxide deficiency by asking the patient to practise voluntary hyperventilation for three minutes.

After forty-five seconds of taking deep, rapid breaths Claire felt so light-headed and tired that she had to stop. I told her that if forty-five seconds of overbreathing made her feel so unwell, I could imagine how ill she must feel when she breathed like that all the time.

Because switching from chest breathing to diaphragmatic breathing can be so difficult, I asked her to come again with a twenty-minute appointment the following week in order to do some more work on her problem. In the meantime I asked her to practise diaphragmatic breathing for at least twenty minutes twice a day; twenty minutes in the morning before getting out of bed and twenty minutes in the evening before going to sleep; as well as at any time when she felt her symptoms were coming on.

By the end of the session, her hoarseness and persistent dry cough had disappeared and so had her daughter's. She looked much calmer and intrigued.

Second Session: Exploring the Feelings

A week later Claire came on her own and started the session by complaining about irrelevant things, such as a little nodule on her cheek. She kept sighing as she was talking and I asked her whether she felt any better since last time. She made a dismissive gesture with her hand and said that she had a lot on her mind.

I urged her to tell me what it was and she said that her father had been admitted to hospital. He had had part of his stomach removed in the past, because of some growths that could have turned nasty. Recently he had been feeling very weak and was admitted for tests. I asked her whether she was close to her father and she said that he used to beat her black and blue and she hated him for that. She was the eldest child and he blamed her for everything.

'What about your mother?', I asked, 'Did she not protect you?'

'She did not dare', Claire said. 'He used to beat her as well.'

When the NSPCC called, her mother would ask Claire not to tell them that it was her father who caused the bruises because they might take her away from home and from her mother. So she used to tell them that she had tumbled downstairs. She used to wish him dead!

'So if he dies in hospital, will you feel guilty about the death wishes that you had as a child?', I asked.

She told me that when she was fourteen years old he fell from a ladder and knocked himself unconscious. When the ambulance came to take him to hospital she remembered saying that she did not mean him to die.

'This means that at the time you were worried in case your death wishes might come true', I commented.

She said that she knew that wishes do not come true.

I suggested that perhaps there was a little bit of her that still believed that they might come true.

She accepted that she did have a guilty conscience about the death wishes that she had towards her father as a child, but she almost simultaneously denied it and felt confused. I encouraged her self-observations and told her that I thought she had put her finger on the problem. I asked her when was the last time that her father beat her and she said that it was just after her wedding when she was eighteen years old. But then, she went on, he is her dad and, despite the past, she loved him. Of late he had changed and had become a caring father who showed his affection and invited her to his home for barbecues. She would like him to live as long as possible, even though she felt that he had robbed her of her childhood. She said that she would like very much to help him now but did not know how.

I suggested that perhaps she would like to take over his illness. She looked at me with tears in her eyes. She had thought that she would like to die in his place. She had had such a terrible childhood – not a childhood at all. As a mother she had lost her temper with her children a few times, had shouted at them and smacked them. The thought of becoming cruel like her father was so painful that she wanted to kill herself. When she married she was praying that her husband did not turn out to be like her father. Fortunately he is a wonderful man: one in a million. Very often she wondered why couldn't her father have been in her childhood the way he is now.

I told her that at the moment the problem was that she felt guilty about the death wishes that she had had for her father as a child. It sounded as though if anything happened to her father now, she would feel responsible for his death. There was still a fourteen-year-old at the back of her mind who still thought that her wishes could come true.

In reply to my comment she said that she had had a dream recently in which she dreamt that her mother died. She woke up screaming and rang home immediately to find out if she was all right.

I took this opportunity to point out to her that even now she is not sure whether her dreams or wishes may come true.

'Don't think I am mad', she said, 'but some dreams have come true. One day I fell asleep reading and I heard voices telling me to look in my children's bedroom. I woke up and went to check and found the bedcovers on fire. The corner of the blanket had touched the electric fire. *I am trying not to think of anything in case it comes true.*'

She said that she did not want to talk about her childhood because the bad feelings were coming back. Then she took out of her handbag a form for a barium swallow that one of my partners had given her in an attempt to investigate her gastrointestinal symptoms. She asked me whether she should go to have the test. Before I had time to answer she tore the form up and said that she did not want to have it done.

'Why not?', I asked; 'Are you afraid of what they might find?'

'No.' she said. 'I am not worth bothering about. I am worthless.'

At the time, her sense of shame took me by surprise and I was at a loss as to how to deal with it in a psychotherapeutic way. So I disagreed with her. I told her that she was a good mother and that it was very important to tell herself that whatever happened to her father, it had nothing to do with her. She could not take his place so that he lived and she died.

She told me that she did not want to see me again because talking about her childhood brought back all the pain.

'On the contrary', I replied. 'Your guilt influences the way you breathe and it is very important to talk about the way you feel. The more you talk about your feelings the less frightening the symptoms will become.'

I invited her to come again with another twenty-minute appointment a week later.

Third Session: Adaptive Conclusion

When she arrived for the third session, she looked much more composed. She said that she felt a lot better since she started practising diaphragmatic breathing. She did not feel so dizzy but she felt breathless at times so that all her symptoms could not be due to her breathing difficulty, she said defiantly.

'But are you breathing correctly?', I asked.

'Of course ! I am breathing exactly as you told me, I am not stupid.'

I asked her to show me, and she lay on the couch and said that she felt very self-conscious. She covered her eyes with her hands and giggled nervously. She said that she felt too nervous to do it when somebody was watching. I encouraged her to try and even though she had made great progress since the first time I examined her, there was still some thoracic breathing. I stressed how difficult diaphragmatic breathing can be at the beginning and that regular practise was needed.

She insisted that all her symptoms could not be due to her breathing, and I pointed out to her that it was her guilt that affected her breathing.

'I do not feel guilty', she said.

I was astonished at her denial. What about last week's session? Had she forgotten it?

I suggested that she might not feel guilty now but she used to when she was a little girl and wished her father dead. As a way of reply she told me another dream. She dreamt that her father died. She was crying in her dream and she ran to tell her mother. Then her father got up and he was well. As soon as she awoke she rang her father to make sure that he was all right.

'There you are', I said. 'This is what the guilt is about. The dream is like the wishes you had had as a little girl. You are still afraid that they might come true.'

She insisted that she did not feel any guilt about her father's illness at the moment but that it was probably at the back of her mind. Then she told me that when she went home after our last session *she thought and thought* until she realised that it was her father who should feel guilty and not her. He was the one who had wrecked her childhood. She used to feel guilty as a child but the guilt belongs to the past.

I told her that it should stay in the past, and asked her whether her father felt guilty.

She did not think so. Her father had told her mother that out of all her sisters and brothers it was her life he made hell and it was she who was the first to help him.

I asked whether he had ever apologised for the misery he caused her and she told me that this was not his style.

As she had improved considerably since I first saw her, I did not give her a further appointment and left it up to her to contact me if she needed to.

Discussion

After I had elicited all Claire's physical symptoms and had understood them as the result of carbon dioxide deficiency, I was able to diminish her physiological arousal by teaching her diaphragmatic breathing. Once the somatic accompaniments of her affects subsided she could direct her attention to their cognitive aspects and talk about them. Since her father's recent admission to hospital, her guilty expectation of punishment for the murderous wishes she has had for him, became accentuated. However, because she was afraid to experience and think about her emotions in case her murderous fantasies came true in a magical omnipotent way, she handled her feelings by not thinking about them and became involved in a vicious circle of hatred and guilt. She also became afraid that the physical symptoms were due to a serious illness – her deserved punishment, perhaps, for her murderous thoughts. She had other feelings as well, such as a longing for a better father, and a particularly painful one which was much less verbalised than the hatred and the guilt. This was the sense of worthlessness that one often finds in abused children. It is as if during the years of abuse an impression is formed that to be treated in this degrading way must mean that they are worthless. She expressed that feeling in a dramatic manner by tearing up the X-ray form in self-loathing. One can understand how such feelings can make patients avoid medical care because they think they are not worth it.

During our conversation, I helped her to identify and name her feelings. This process also challenged the remnants of her primary process thinking, according to which wishes may come true. After this she was able to start thinking about her feelings by herself, despite experiencing mental pain from the reactivation of negative emotions. Finally, she arrived at the adaptive conclusion that the guilty person was the abusing adult and not the abused child.

Denise: The Fear of Dying

A 37-year-old bank clerk who was very thin and had short dark hair walked into the surgery one day without an appointment, wanting to be seen as an emergency. She requested an extension of her sick leave because she did not think that her chest infection had cleared and did not feel ready to return to work. I asked her to describe her symptoms to me and she told me that she had a terrible cough and a dry throat, and when she started coughing it went on and on until she felt sick. Then she panicked because she could not catch her breath and felt she might choke.

I asked if she had any more symptoms and she volunteered that she had a tight feeling in the chest. I asked her to describe this feeling a little more accurately. She added that she could only breathe in a little amount. She kept trying to take deep breaths and it felt like a 'horrible tightness' in her chest and her throat became dry. I asked whether she slept well at night and she said that she woke up after a couple of hours with a tickly throat and a tight chest and started coughing. She managed to go back to sleep but sometimes she woke up again with the same symptoms at around 3 o'clock in the morning. She had also been feeling very tired, her abdominal and chest muscles felt achy, she felt dizzy and light-headed at times and she was yawning a lot. She wondered whether her symptoms had anything to do with giving up smoking, but as she had given up smoking once before without any symptoms it was rather unlikely. Then she wondered whether her symptoms might have anything to do with stress? I asked what the stress might be and she told me that three weeks previously, her place of work in the City had been totally destroyed by a massive explosion caused by a bomb. When she visited the scene of destruction a few days later and saw the devastation, she went into a state of shock. She realised that if the bomb had exploded during a weekday she would have been killed. Soon after that, her symptoms started with a tickly cough. She described all this in a quiet, reserved manner, but I could sense her fear behind the detached faint smile.

I proceeded to examine her. I checked her blood pressure, measured her PEFR and listened to her chest. Everything was normal. I asked her to lie on the couch and observed her breathing pattern, which was obviously upper thoracic. I told her that I did not think she had a chest infection, but rather that her symptoms were due to carbon dioxide deficiency brought on by the way she breathed. I explained hyperventilation syndrome and taught her how to breathe with the diaphragm, as I have already described in Claire's case history. She found diaphragmatic breathing very difficult and I invited her to come again the following week with a double appointment for more breathing retraining and emotion coaching.

When she came back a week later she told me that she had been practising diaphragmatic breathing. This had helped to take the sense of suffocation away, but she was not back to normal. She was still coughing, had an ache between her shoulder blades and her throat was still dry. She still had the chest tightness and woke up at around 3 o'clock in the morning coughing, and vomiting at the end of a coughing bout.

I wondered whether the persistent physical symptoms could be maintained by the continuing physiological arousal of unacknowledged emotions and I asked her to tell me again what she felt like when she went to her workplace and saw the devastation.

She repeated that when she went to have a look four days after the explosion and saw that everything was destroyed, she went into a state of shock. The thought occurred to her that if the bomb had gone off during the week, she would have been killed because the desk where she worked was totally destroyed. She thought that if she had been killed, her children would have been left without a mother.

When I asked about her own mother's health, she told me that she was healthy, but not her mother's sister. She had had an operation for carcinoma of the ovary one month before the explosion and they were told that ovarian cancer runs in families. Her grandmother died of cancer of the ovary ten years previously and her mother is under observation for an ovarian cyst. Denise had had menstrual irregularities last year ... She left her sentence unfinished, not daring to draw the conclusion.

'So are you worried that if the bomb does not get you, the ovarian cancer will?', I asked. She told me that one of my partners had already referred her for a gynaecological appointment, but she had not heard from the hospital yet. In the same breath she said that it was stupid to worry about these things; she should push them to the back of her mind and get on with her work. But then she appreciated that she would feel easier in her mind if she knew that there was nothing wrong with her.

I said that it was perfectly understandable to worry about having cancer of the ovary in her circumstances. The destruction she had witnessed must have brought the fear of dying to the front of her mind. I promised to arrange an urgent gynaecological appointment and asked her to come and see me again the following week.

When she arrived she told me that she felt a lot better, but she was still coughing a little. I sensed that unless her fear of dying from cancer was lifted, her symptoms would not improve. She told me that when she saw the devastation of her workplace by the bomb she had become aware of her fear that she might die. However, it was only when she talked to me that she became aware that it was not the bomb that she was afraid of, but the cancer. Another bomb, so to speak, ticking in her ovaries. She felt that even if they had to take her uterus and ovaries out, she would not mind if it meant living without the fear of developing ovarian cancer.

Following this conversation I arranged an urgent appointment with the gynaecologist, with whom I discussed her fears. A few weeks later I learned that she had had a laparoscopic biopsy for a tubal lesion shown on ultrasound. The result was negative for cancer but in view of her family history she was to be offered long-term follow-up in a special clinic.

Discussion

When Denise saw the destruction caused by the bomb, she must have unconsciously equated her death with the devastation of her workplace and she had anticipated a premature absurd and unacceptable death. The fear that she might have been killed in the explosion and might have left her children motherless overshadowed briefly a more realistic fear that her own mother and she herself might die of cancer of the ovary, so that both she and her own children might be left motherless. This fear was so strong that it threatened to overwhelm her and was expressed in physical symptoms. Her preoccupation with these distracted her from becoming aware of the real danger and encouraged the development of a phobic avoidance of her workplace (Lazarus and Kostan 1969).

However, after I had helped her to reduce the intensity of her physical symptoms, she became able to discover and tolerate her fear of dying from cancer of the ovary, so that we could talk about it openly. This led to the adaptive action and realistic management of her gynaecological problem.

CONCLUSION

I understand hyperventilation syndrome to be the consequence of a maladaptive behaviour in which patients handle their affects in a certain way that leads to a vicious circle. It would appear that at least three affective states underlie the irregular upper thoracic breathing that causes carbon dioxide deficiency: an affect that threatens to overwhelm the patient, primary anxiety about having this affect, and secondary anxiety about the significance of the carbon dioxide deficiency symptoms. Upper thoracic breathing is their undifferentiated non-specific motor expression.

The aim of my treatment is to break this vicious circle by addressing all three affective states in six consecutive steps, starting from the most easily accessible secondary anxiety and working towards the original threatening affect.

A most important feature of my work is the use of physical touch in order to regulate patients' breathing and change it from an emergency upper thoracic pattern to a relaxing diaphragmatic pattern. This approach creates in a direct and immediate way an atmosphere of trust and safety. It also minimises the intensity of the frightening physical symptoms and gives patients a sense of control over their bodies.

In the safety of this new environment there is much more chance for patients not only to identify but also to verbalise their affects. In this way feelings may be synthesised from their purely physical components to become a psychological experience. Once patients become aware of their feelings they should be in a position to take better care of themselves.

6 PSYCHOSOMATIC ASPECTS OF ASTHMA

WHAT IS ASTHMA?

Asthma is a medical condition that is often confused with hyperventilation. Although the mechanism of breathlessness is different from that of hyperventilation, the two conditions may coexist and the management of asthma can benefit significantly from correcting the upper chest breathing pattern which is also part of the treatment of hyperventilation (Thomas et al. 2001).

Asthma causes episodes of breathlessness. These are not continuous, but consist of intermittent attacks. They are due to narrowing of the breathing tubes inside the lungs, which is due in turn to spasm of the muscle that surrounds the bronchial tubes, swelling of the mucosal lining and blockage by excessive secretion of mucus by the mucosal lining, or by a combination of all three.

WHAT IS THE CAUSE OF ASTHMA?

Asthma is caused by unusual irritability of the airways, which may react to many stimuli by spasm of the muscle that surrounds them, swelling of the mucosal lining and excessive mucus production.

The main triggers of asthma are allergy, infection and emotion. Interaction of the biological and emotional factors are usually responsible.

An example is given by Trousseau, a famous nineteenth-century French physician who was an asthmatic. His worst attack occurred in a grain loft. The air was dusty, but on this occasion there was an emotional charge in the atmosphere. Trousseau suspected his coachman of dishonesty in measuring the oats and had decided on this occasion to supervise the operation. He had been exposed to an atmosphere of dust a hundred times before. But this time the dust acted on him while he was in a peculiar state. His nervous system was shaken by the influence of emotion caused by the suspicion of theft, however trifling, committed by one of his servants. It is interesting to note that Trousseau's account does not go as far as naming the emotion he writes about. This difficulty in using language to identify and name emotions may be a vulnerability factor in psychosomatic patients as discussed earlier.

In the present anti-emotional climate of British culture you will seldom hear a reference to the interaction of emotional and biological factors in asthma. This is particularly true of popular publications on asthma. In a recent article in the *Reader's Digest*, with the title 'Asthma alert', the author gives a long list of allergic triggers, such as air pollution, ground level ozone, thunderstorms, which help release allergens in the pollen; smoking, house dust mites, and even volcanic dust in the atmosphere – but not a word about the emotions. However, reading between the lines it is possible to detect a certain dissatisfaction with the attitude of parents to their children's asthma. The author calls it ignorance. When it comes to medication, he writes, parents are not always a child's best friends. Parents, the article concludes, need to understand more about the causes and treatment of asthma. (In our relationship to our patients very often we stand for the parents.) Unfortunately the author means allergic causes and pharmacological treatment only. I believe that by not calling attention to the relevance of emotional factors, such publications miss an opportunity to educate patients about aspects of their personality which can interfere with the correct management of their asthma.

In fact, the clearest evidence that psychological factors can precipitate asthmatic attacks comes from learning experiments. Luparello, in an experiment that might not be considered ethical nowadays, compared asthmatic patients and normal controls. He gave everybody saline solution to inhale and told them that it was a solution of a substance that the asthmatic patients knew could precipitate asthma. Of all the participants only the asthmatic patients showed a significant rise in airway resistance, a simple measure of air tube irritability, and became breathless. Then he gave them saline solution to inhale, telling them that it was an asthmatic reliever. Within minutes the asthma improved (Luparello et al. 1968).

Asthmatic attacks can also be conditioned. Groen wrote about an asthmatic Dutch woman known to be allergic to pollens and house dust mites, who believed herself to be allergic to goldfish!

This seemed rather strange, since there is no way a goldfish could give rise to allergens that could be inhaled. Under circumstances where lung function tests could be carried out, she was shown a live goldfish in a bowl. She immediately became wheezy. On a second occasion she was shown a toy goldfish in a bowl. Despite the fact that she realised it was ridiculous, she again became wheezy. Finally she became wheezy when shown an empty goldfish bowl (Groen and Pelser 1960).

During the course of these tests she had a dream in which she saw a huge goldfish bowl. On a shelf high above it were her books. She wanted to find out why goldfish cause asthma. She climbed on a chair and reached for the book but it was too high. She lost her balance and fell into the goldfish bowl. The fish swam around, she gasped for breath. Her neck became caught in a strand of weed. Suddenly she was awake, wheezing and fighting for breath.

The patient described how, when she was a child, her mother had thrown away her goldfish which she had loved very much and had saved her pocket money to buy. The memories became all too real when, in an attempt to stop the wheezing in the final study, the experimenter smashed the goldfish bowl. The wheezing became worse. 'This is exactly what my mother did', she explained. 'She threw the bowl into the dustbin.'

This is also a reminder that mother–child interaction is often the determining factor in asthma.

HOW DO PATIENTS PRESENT?

When the airways narrow, more effort is required to achieve a satisfactory flow of air. The increased effort produces the sense of breathing difficulty. In asthma there is more difficulty in breathing out than breathing in. The patient usually complains of chest tightness, cough and wheeze. It is not so much the symptoms themselves as the circumstances under which they occur that makes asthma so readily recognisable.

Tightness in the chest, a congested cough and wheezing occur in paroxysms. These may be very brief episodes of chest tightness lasting a matter of minutes, or more prolonged episodes of wheezing lasting up to an hour or so, which may merge into a full-blown attack of asthma.

As I mentioned earlier, the most important characteristic of asthma is the extreme sensitivity of the airways to irritant stimuli. Cold air, fumes of petrol, gas fire, wood smoke and cigarette smoke can cause chest tightness; violent movements of the chest such as coughing or laughing can set up a short paroxysm of wheezing. Irregular upper chest movements associated with hyperventilation syndrome can also bring on an asthmatic attack.

But the best documented stimulus that can set off a prolonged episode of wheezing is exercise. Unlike the rest of us who can become breathless during exercise and recover as soon as the exercise stops, the asthmatic becomes even more short of breath. Instead of being able to relax and get his breath back, he becomes wheezy and breathless and he may not recover for half an hour.

Apparently some forms of exercise can cause worse asthma than others. Swimming is the least harmful and running is the worst exercise. Six to eight minutes of free running is recommended when testing for exercise induced asthma. Many asthmatics become wheezy in less time.

Another characteristic of asthma is that many patients become breathless and wheezy in the small hours of the morning. This phenomenon has become known as the 'morning dip'.

Before an attack, there may also be premonitory symptoms such as heaviness of the chest or sluggishness to one's accustomed work. Many patients describe mood changes, often irritability, or apprehension which is difficult to explain. Hippocrates was the first doctor to observe that the asthmatic guards himself against anger. Yet any intense emotional arousal may precipitate or accompany an asthmatic attack. Humiliation, fear, anxiety, longing, grief, guilt may be related to the onset of an attack. Adult patients are frequently depressed and moody. This complex emotional state can occur in the intervals between or during attacks. Yet patients very rarely make a link between their feelings and previous possible precipitants such as loss, longing or disappointment.

DIAGNOSIS

A doctor who elicits the circumstances in which the symptoms occur will immediately think of asthma. He will of course wish to confirm the diagnosis by examining the patient physically and by doing a simple test.

The typical findings on listening to the chest with a stethoscope are a prolonged breathing-out phase and high-pitched whistling sounds that we call wheezes. The test is measurement of the Peak Expiratory Flow Rate (PEFR) with the peak flow meter, a simple device into which the subject blows and which locks when the peak value has been reached. Providing you put as much effort into the blow as you can, then how fast you blow will depend on whether your breathing tubes are wide or narrow. If they have become narrowed because of asthma, it will be more difficult to blow out. So the peak flow value will be less than when the breathing tubes are wide open. Peak flow is a useful measure of the severity of asthma.

HOW COMMON IS ASTHMA?

Asthma is very common. Its prevalence at the moment is considered to be around 5 per cent.This means that in a typical practice of 10000 patients there will be approximately 500 current asthmatics, some of whom may not have been diagnosed (Pearson 1990).

Asthma may start in childhood or in middle age. Also, despite the definition of asthma as intermittent attacks of breathlessness, it can be continuous or persistent. Asthmatic patients with continuous chronic asthma have a worse prognosis.

It is important to remember that children may present with coughing alone without any wheezing being obvious. Because of this, the doctor may not immediately think of asthma. However, a careful history of the circumstances under which the coughing occurs will reveal that it follows the same pattern as that described for the wheezing: it will be more obvious during the night, on waking up in the morning and after exercise.

MORTALITY/INTRACTABILITY

Despite recent advances in pharmacology, the number of patients who are dying of asthma has not decreased. In the UK, 2,000 patients die of asthma each year. Fifty of those are children aged under fifteen years. The British Thoracic Association has issued guidelines about the management of asthma in order to improve the doctor's response to the asthmatic patient. Unfortunately, and sometimes to their cost, the majority of asthmatics suffer and tolerate too much without complaint. They are also reluctant to call their GP for help. Anthony Storr, a psychoanalyst who was also an asthmatic, used to boast that he never allowed anyone to call the doctor until he was so breathless that he could no longer speak but had to communicate in writing (Lane and Storr 1981).

Because of the potentially lethal consequences of the asthmatic behaviour, this has for many years been the object of intensive study. Even though there is no such thing as a uniform asthmatic personality type, there is some consensus that asthmatics are overcontrolled and tend to bottle up their emotions. Lask conducted an interesting study of asthma patients in general practice. He found that, contrary to his expectations, the majority of asthmatics shared an attitude of independence and reluctance to seek help. They managed their illness alone and did not like to confide. The asthmatics who were demanding and used their illness as an excuse for getting attention and summoning the doctor were a minority 15 per cent of the adult asthmatic population (Lask 1966). Anthony Storr thought that this finding might be interpreted as evidence that asthmatics are essentially rather dependent people, but are reluctant to admit or to give in to this aspect of their personalities. These extremes of behaviour – the independent attitude, on the one hand; and the demanding behaviour, on the other, have become the object of research by Dicks and colleagues (Dicks et al. 1977).

Dicks developed a panic-fear scale that differentiated asthmatics according to the frequency with which they report panic and fear symptoms during asthmatic attacks. Patients scoring extremely highly on the panic-fear scale are characterised as fearful and emotionally labile. They profess to have their feelings hurt more easily than others, to feel helpless and to give up easily when there are difficulties.

Patients whose score is very low describe themselves as experiencing little discomfort; they deny the presence of anxiety and claim to be unusually calm and self-controlled. About 35–40 per cent of asthmatic patients treated at the National Jewish Hospital and research centre in Denver, Colorado, fall into one of these two categories.

A very interesting observation that has great implications for treatment was that patients with the most panic-fear symptoms were those discharged on the most intensive oral medication. Further, they were not necessarily those with the worst objectively measured pulmonary function. In other words, their doctor's decision to give the strongest steroids was not based on objective measurement of their pulmonary function but was influenced by the patient's emotional display. Another interesting observation was that patients with high panic-fear scores stayed in hospital twice as long as the low scorers. Both high and low scorers were readmitted twice as frequently as those with moderate scores.

According to Dicks, the therapeutic implications of his research are that both high and low scorers can be helped by attempting to modify their behaviour.

The high scorers can learn to perceive that they are not as powerless as they think. They can develop appropriate strategies of personal control over their illness and over the ways in which they react to illness. It is also important to help them recognise how they use their illness to achieve a dependent relationship.

Low-scoring patients may be helped by modifying their techniques of denial and counterdependency. This is particularly relevant where denial of symptoms has resulted in poor compliance with medical treatment and avoidance of doctors.

Psychoanalytically oriented investigations of small numbers of asthmatic patients have provided a way of understanding hidden contradictory attitudes and feelings which are not obvious when one only observes the behaviour. French and Alexander sought to provide a specific psychological account of the conflicts which play a role in asthma. They proposed what is known as the nuclear conflict theory of asthma, which they believed to be true for all asthmatics.

They proposed as the fundamental dynamic structure of asthmatic disorder, a deep dependence on a mother figure plus the fear of becoming estranged from her by offending her, not only by desiring her sexually but also by favouring one's own interests over the mother's security and pleasure (Alexander and French 1946).

The mother was felt to be a person who held the child closely and at the same time would be alienated by the child's urges either for intense closeness or separation. They conceived of the asthmatic attack as a manifestation of suppressed crying which helped to re-establish the union of the child to its caring mother.

Deutsch (1953), Fenichel (1945) and Sperling (1963) suggested that rather than a particular set of emotions being responsible for asthma, conflicting fantasies related to both primitive impulses and inhibitory forces were communicated in body language. This hypothesis states that asthma represents a conversion, in the psychological sense, of a conflict into learned, symbolically relevant somatic expressive patterns. Evidence for this theory comes from clinical reports, such as Lofgren's, of a patient whose asthma cleared on recovering memories of a traumatic strangling scene in childhood (Lofgren 1961).

Knapp has formulated the more comprehensive hypothesis that asthma results when there is simultaneous activation of powerful threatening impulses, and efforts to inhibit these. A prior condition is that both these elements should have become channelled by biologic and learned predisposition into expression via pulmonary dysfunction. This hypothesis fits a general view of the developmental history of many asthmatics. It would see them as having an often quite circumscribed 'psychosomatic lesion', so to speak, capable of coexisting with highly adaptive and gifted personality features (Knapp 1989).

A particular result is a persisting attachment to a parental, especially maternal figure, toward whom they have a dependent, often seductively tinged relationship.

Detailed biographical material from a celebrated asthmatic, Marcel Proust supports this hypothesis. The dominant manifest theme of his life and work was his attachment to his adored *maman*, and in many ways his profound identification with her. He never ceased mourning her death, which precipitated a depression requiring hospitalisation. Before his own death, he openly longed for reunion with her in the same grave. Yet he moved her furniture into a Paris brothel where he indulged in his private, perverse, sadistic and masochistic activities. His need to keep his rebellious and angry impulses tamed was illustrated in a letter to his mother. After one of his frequent intense quarrels with her he spent the night in an asthmatic exacerbation. The next day he wrote to her: 'I would rather have asthma and please you' (Hayman 1990). Of all the statements about asthma, I find this the most profound.

Problems in the relationship between mother and child may be responsible for the intractable asthma that occurs in 10 per cent of all children who have asthma. Fifty per cent of these children improve when they are taken away from home.

Abramson has commented in several papers on the beneficial effects of removing the child from his family environment to a hospital or camp, and has called this 'parentectomy' (Abramson and Peshkin 1961).

Minuchin, a family therapist, and his collaborators studied the families of children whose recurrent and severe attacks represented an exacerbation of asthma in response to emotional arousal. They called these 'psychosomatic families' and discovered that their functioning differed markedly from that of the families of normal asthmatics, and identified a cluster of four transactional patterns felt to be characteristic of a family process that encourages somatisation (Minuchin et al. 1978). These are enmeshment, overprotectiveness, rigidity, and lack of conflict resolution.

1. *Enmeshment* refers to a situation where the family members are intrusive and over-involved with one another. The effect of this transactional pattern is a decrease in the autonomy and privacy of each individual.
2. *Overprotectiveness* results in a decrease in extrafamilial relationships and activities.
3. *Rigidity* refers to the parents' denial of the need to change. When a child in an effectively functioning family reaches adolescence, his family can change the rules and transactional patterns in ways that allow for increased autonomy appropriate to age, while still preserving family continuity. But the family of a psychosomatically ill child insists on retaining the accustomed methods of interaction.
4. *Lack of Conflict Resolution* results from total concentration on the patient's symptoms which enables the parents to avoid dealing with their own marital conflicts. A consequence is the development of a dysfunctional set, a pattern of defective or ineffective communication between two or more people that results in lack of resolution of disagreements and the perpetuation of stress and tension.

Minuchin has developed a family therapy approach as an alternative to parentectomy for the treatment of severe intractable asthma in childhood. Parentectomy is considered to be a process that is emotionally traumatic for the family and the patient. To the family it implies that it has a harmful influence on the patient and amplifies the feelings of hopelessness that pervade the entire family. In the patient it crystallises the formation of a profound negative self-image as a defective, sick, helpless person. The child has become a medical invalid crippled by his symptoms. Family therapy enables the child to stay with his family. It changes the structure and functioning of the family to eliminate the factors reinforcing the symptoms and help the patient to grow and develop in an age-appropriate fashion.

THERAPEUTIC CONSIDERATIONS

Besides medical treatment, many psychological treatments have been used in an effort to help asthmatic patients. Behaviour therapy, psychotherapy, psychoanalysis, family therapy, group therapy and also hypnosis are all claimed to be successful.

However, it must always be borne in mind that despite modern advances in treatment the mortality of asthma has not decreased. This must mean that there is something better that can be done. At a simple clinical level, the management of asthmatic patients becomes easier if the therapist takes into account the typical aspects of the personality traits and attitudes.

Paulley has drawn attention to the fact that asthmatics have a typical sensitivity to domination and rejection (Paulley and Pelser 1989). He found that they are sensitive to smothering, both physical and emotional, and they react to touching as an intrusion equal to smothering. They are especially sensitive to people behaving in an authoritarian way. This sensitivity originates in childhood in response to parental behaviour or even tone of voice. A common experience for many asthmatics is that their parents did not believe that their coughing bouts in childhood were due to real illness: they reacted to them with derision and irritability, as if they were acts of insubordination or malingering. If given the opportunity, asthmatic patients will admit their intense dislike of anything they see as domination or being pushed about. They may also react visibly and audibly with changes in posture and breathing and by coughing in response to such threats. High-pitched, sharp comments are particularly resented as replays of childhood experiences of a parent and result in audible wheezing within a minute or two. Asthmatics are also vulnerable to beating or the threat of beating, a fairly common experience in many. My first asthmatic patient was a man who developed asthma in middle age after he was beaten up by a group of men who mistook him for somebody else.

Paulley points out that asthmatics have in addition a typical sensitivity to rejection. This also originates in childhood, but the rejection is often provoked by the asthmatic's own behaviour, albeit unconsciously. Asthmatic children are often considered to be precocious and this may annoy others. In adults the same behaviour is seen as cockiness. They like to challenge or contradict and in this way court the rejection which at the same time they so much dislike. For example, a doctor may suggest a new inhaler which he has found useful. The patient may reply: 'Ah, but I have tried it already doctor and it was of no use to me.'

The therapeutic implication of these observations is that in our encounters with asthmatic patients we must take care to behave in a way that does not appear oppressive or dominating. We must avoid touching them or giving commands in loud voices or even standing too close to them.

A doctor who does not reject his patient, however strong the provocation, may be the first person in an asthmatic's life who is tested and who does not react aggressively. Recognition of this sensitivity to domination and rejection has led many hospital units to adopt an open door policy according to which asthmatics are encouraged to come in whenever they feel ill, stay as long as they need to and leave when they feel ready. This policy makes them feel secure from an anticipation of rejection when they turn up in Casualty.

ASTHMA AND HYPERVENTILATION SYNDROME

There is a reciprocal relationship between asthma and hyperventilation syndrome. Not only can the latter trigger asthma in susceptible individuals, but it can also complicate asthma and contribute to its intractability. Liebman and Minuchin, in their paper 'The use of structural family therapy in the treatment of intractable asthma', have reported on the treatment of seven children with intractable asthma who were helped considerably by the use of family therapy which prevented them from having acute attacks requiring hospital treatment. (Liebman et al. 1974). They described how their team encouraged the fathers of these children to help them decrease the intensity and frequency of their acute asthmatic attacks by teaching them to practise diaphragmatic breathing at the first sign of bronchocon-striction. Although these exercises were not sufficient to prevent relapses in the context of a dysfunctional family system, they did enable the patients to abort acute attacks and decrease their symptoms.

THE BUTEYKO TECHNIQUE

Professor Konstantin Buteyko, a Russian doctor, has come to the conclusion that asthma is in fact caused by hyperventilation. As far back as 1953 in a paper entitled 'The biochemical basis of K.P.Buteyko's theory of the disease of deep respiration', he discussed the biological mechanisms by which deep upper respiratory breathing can precipitate or complicate asthma leading to maintenance of the disease. He went on to develop a series of special breathing exercises, techniques and lifestyle changes that are taught over a minimum of five consecutive one hour daily sessions. These exercises emphasise the importance of diaphragmatic breathing and result in the ability to overcome asthma attacks by restoring a normal level of carbon dioxide which allows the bronchial tubes to dilate.

The Buteyko technique became popular in Australia, where the incidence of asthma is high and the Australian Buteyko Association was formed in

1994 (Ameisen, P. J. 1997). Because the claims of successful treatment, carried out by Buteyko practitioners, have provoked a very sceptical response, to say the least, from the medical establishment, a group of interested physicians and Buteyko practitioners set up a number of clinical trials the best known of which is the Queensland one. The study, flawed as it might be, provides the best evidence to date about the effectiveness of the Buteyko technique. It compared the response of a group of asthma patients who were coached in the Buteyko breathing technique with that of a similar group who were given standard asthma education physiotherapy classes and relaxation exercises. The trial concluded that the patients who were practising the Buteyko breathing technique reduced their hyperventilation and their use of beta2 agonist inhalers. A trend toward reduced inhaled steroid use and better quality of life was observed in these patients without objective changes in measures of airway calibre (Bowler, S. et al. 1998).

Although it may be an oversimplification to view asthma as the body's defence against the falling levels of carbon dioxide there is good physiological evidence that overbreathing can trigger constriction of almost any of the body's smooth muscle tubing (i.e.: bowel, bronchi, arteries) by altering the relationship of calcium and magnesium ions and the balance between sympathetic and parasympathetic activity when the body is ripe for the triggering.

It is important therefore to say that although the Buteyko technique has a place in the management of asthma it must not be seen as an alternative to pharmacological treatment but rather as an element of education for health and performance that should be available to all asthmatic patients.

7 AN EXAMPLE OF ADAPTIVE RESPONSE TO POSITIVE EMOTIONS AND ITS THERAPEUTIC POTENTIAL
Some Thoughts on a Case of Asthma Described by Donald Winnicott

Donald Winnicott had been observing infants in his paediatric clinic at the Paddington Green Children's Hospital for twenty years. In a large number of cases he recorded in minute detail the way infants behaved in a familiar setting which he staged within the ordinary clinic routine and which he called the set situation.

Mothers and their children waited in the passage outside a fairly large room in which he worked and the exit of one mother and child was the signal for the entrance of the next. He had chosen a large room because so much could be seen and done in the time that it took the mother and her child to reach him from the door at the opposite end of the room. By the time the mother reached him he had made contact with her and probably with the child as well by his expression, and he had had time to remember the case if it was not a new patient.

When the mother was holding a baby he would ask her to sit opposite him, with the angle of the table coming between him and her as she sat down with the baby on her knee. He routinely placed a right-angled shining tongue depressor at the edge of the table, inviting the mother to place the child in such a way that if he should wish to handle the spatula, he could do so.

Ordinarily a mother would understand what Winnicott was about, and he could easily and gradually describe to her that there was to be a period of time in which she and he would contribute as little as possible, so that what happened could fairly be put down to the child's initiative. In this setting the mother showed by her ability or relative inability to follow his suggestions something of what she was like at home. If she was anxious about infection or had strong feelings against putting things into the mouth, if she was hasty or moved impulsively, these characteristics would be shown up.

THE INFANT'S BEHAVIOUR

Winnicott described a normal sequence of events and he held that any variation from this was significant.

- Stage I: The baby, who is inevitably *interested* in this new attractive object, puts his hand to the spatula, but at this moment he hesitates. He looks at Winnicott and then at his mother with big eyes and watches and waits, holding his body still. In some cases he withdraws interest completely and buries his face in his mother's bosom.
- Stage 2: During this period of hesitation the baby holds his body still. Gradually he becomes brave enough to let his feelings develop. His mouth becomes flabby and full of saliva. Before long he puts the spatula into his mouth and draws it with his gums. The baby now seems to feel that the spatula is in his possession. He bangs it on the table or else he holds it to Winnicott's or the mother's mouth and looks very pleased if they pretend to be fed by it.
- Stage 3: The baby first drops the spatula as if by mistake. When it is given back to him he is pleased, plays with it again and drops it once more but this time less by mistake. When it is given to him again he drops it on purpose and thoroughly enjoys aggressively getting rid of it. This situation is normal for babies between the ages of five and fifteen months.

CASE PRESENTATION

In a famous paper 'The observation of infants in a set situation', Winnicott described the case of a baby girl called Margaret who developed and emerged out of an attack of asthma while under observation (Winnicott 1975b).

Margaret, a seven-month-old baby, was brought to his clinic by her mother because the night before the consultation she had been wheezing all night. The mother herself developed asthma when she became pregnant with Margaret, whose older sister was seven months old. She was bad until one month before the consultation. Since then she had had no asthma. The relationship between mother and Margaret was good and she was feeding at the breast satisfactorily. Winnicott's observations of Margaret who developed asthma on two occasions in this familiar set situation gives us an opportunity to discuss the emotional context within which the symptoms developed.

The symptoms of asthma did not come unheralded. Mother reported that for three days Margaret had been stirring in her sleep, only sleeping for ten minutes at a time, waking and screaming and trembling. For a month she had been putting her fists to her mouth and this had recently become somewhat compulsive and anxious. For three days she had had a slight cough, but the wheezing only became definite the night before the consultation.

At the beginning of the consultation the baby sat on mother's lap with the table between them and Winnicott. Mother held the baby round the chest with both hands supporting her body. The child was *interested* in the spatula. She looked at it, she looked at Winnicott and gave him a long steady look with big eyes and sighs. For five minutes she was unable to make up her mind to take the spatula. When she finally did so she could not decide whether to put it into her mouth or not. The wheezing occurred over the period in which the child hesitated about taking it. After the period of hesitation she put it into her mouth and enjoyed the experience.

In the second consultation, a week later, Margaret reached out to take the spatula but again hesitated and the asthma returned. Only gradually she became able to mouth and enjoy the spatula with *confidence*. She was more eager in her mouthing of it than she had been at the previous occasion and made noises while chewing it. She soon dropped it deliberately, and on it being restored she played with it with *excitement*, making a noise while looking at mother and Winnicott, obviously pleased and kicking. She played about and then threw down the spatula. When it was returned to her she put it into her mouth and made wild movements with her hands and then began to be *interested* in other objects, that were near her.

On both occasions the asthma occurred over the period in which the child *hesitated* about taking the spatula. She put her hand to the spatula and then as she controlled her body, her hand and her environment, she developed asthma which involves an involuntary control of expiration. At the moment when she came to feel *confident* about the spatula which was at her mouth, when saliva flowed, when stillness changed to the enjoyment of activity and when watching changed to *self-confidence*, at this moment the asthma ceased A fortnight later the child had no asthma, except for the two attacks in the two consultations. But the mother had redeveloped it. Two months after the consultation the child had no asthma, although of course she was still liable to it.

Because Winnicott was observing the baby under known conditions, it was possible to see that for this child asthma was associated with the moment at which there was *hesitation* or in other words doubt or lack of confidence. According to Winnicott hesitation implies mental conflict. An impulse has been aroused, but temporarily controlled. The asthma coincided on both occasions with the period of control.

The close association between bronchial spasm and anxiety justified the supposition that there was a close relationship between the two.

However, Winnicott goes further and explores the reason that made the baby hesitate after she first became interested in the spatula. He argues that the infant may have learnt to expect the mother to disapprove or even to be angry whenever she handles or mouths something. But whether the mother's attitude determines the baby's behaviour or not, the hesitation means that the infant expects to produce an angry and perhaps revengeful mother by her actions. In order to feel threatened by a truly and obviously angry mother she must have in mind the notion of such an angry mother. The something which the anxiety is about is, in the child's mind, an idea of potential evil, or strictness, and anything that is in the infant's mind can be projected into the novel situation. When there has been no experience of prohibition, the hesitation implies the existence of a fantasy corresponding to another baby's memory of her really strict mother. In either case she has first to curb the impulse to express her interest in handling and mouthing the spatula and only becomes able to allow the impulse to develop again in so far as her testing of the environment shows that it is safe to do so.

Although Winnicott's observations are timeless, he was strongly influenced at the time (1941) by the ideas of Melanie Klein. He understood the dangerous impulse to be the infant's desire to reach in and take something from the mother's body. The baby is afraid that she cannot satisfy her greed without rousing anger and dissatisfaction in her mother. The breathing out might have been felt by the baby to be dangerous if linked to a dangerous idea such as reaching in to take. So control of the impulse comes to be associated with control of breathing out.

ANOTHER WAY OF LOOKING AT THE DANGEROUS IMPULSE

I would like to propose a somewhat different explanation which is based on Winnicott's subsequent work, as well as the work of Ferenczi, Rank and the affect theorist Silvan Tomkins. These researchers have helped us recognise the importance of the positive emotion *interest-excitement* in shaping the child's behaviour in addition to sexual desire and greed. (Excitement can be coassembled with sexual desire and other drives.)

A great part of the time spent with young children requires adults to help them do things they want to do but are not yet competent to do with success or satisfaction. We must not forget that an impulse is an affect bursting to be expressed in action; each child's interest-excitement about the world is elaborated into a unique constellation of preferred activities. All children require matching enthusiasm from an adult to enable them fully to elaborate their preferences into an acceptable version of themselves, so that they can contribute to a self-representation that feels real and can be held on to whenever they meet future rejections by others.

The concept of interest-excitement allows us to understand the child's emotionally complicated breaking-free from maternal embeddedness and the completion of the fundamental task for each person. This task is to establish oneself as a subject rather than simply as an object of another's subjectivity. The performance of this task not only always entails anxiously risking the security of the *status quo* established with others, but also inevitably evokes guilt. This results from the intrinsic favouring of one's own interest-excitement over the group's security and pleasure, symbolically a withdrawal of love from the mother to invest in the self. What we must be willing to endure in order to elaborate our interest-excitement into a communication or an event is the guilt of disrupting the *status quo* of the other. This is always an act of emotional violence to the symbolic mother, even if the intent is not to do violence but simply to act on one's own interest-excitement and enthusiasm. (Spezzano 1993).

The mother's reaction to the child's gestures of autonomy will be decisive for his subsequent progress towards independence. Donald Nathanson has written eloquently about the emotions involved in this process:

A parent who greets with pleasure the burgeoning independence of a child will reinforce the link between that group of skills and childhood pride.

One who experiences the same skills as a threat, or who sees danger in these actions will convey this information to the child in the form of some negative affect, such as fear, anger, distress, disgust, or even shame. The face of negative affect will be a daunting impediment to the child's expectation of the rewarding smile of parental enjoyment. So parents who for their own reasons are made unhappy by childhood independence, will foster the link of independence with shame, the painful affect triggered by any impediment to ongoing positive affect. Any child who grows up with a mother who is frightened and angry about matters of autonomy will be liable to develop a peculiar emotional state in which the affects of shame and fear are bound together and linked to the idea of independence. Since shame affect works to interfere with our ability to get in touch with the object of our interest or enjoyment, it is an intrinsic instrument of isolation and withdrawal. (Nathanson 1992, p. 181)

I believe that in Margaret's case the hesitation or doubt was probably just as much about her lack of confidence concerning whether her interest in the spatula would be recognised and respected, as it was about her fear that her greed might arouse anger in her mother.

Winnicott felt that in the course of making his observations he also brought about some changes in the direction of health. His adaptive response to the child's expression of interest in the spatula offered to the child the experience of daring to want and to take the spatula and making it her own without offending the stability of the immediate environment. This experience acted as a kind of object lesson and had therapeutic value for the infant. At the age which he was considering and all through childhood such an experience is not merely temporarily reassuring. The cumulative effect of happy experiences and of a stable and happy atmosphere round the child is to build up his confidence in people and in the external world and his general feelings of security. The child's belief in the good things and relationships inside himself is also strengthened. Such little steps in the solution of the central problems come in the everyday life of the infant and young child, and every time the problem is solved, something is added to the child's stability and the foundations of emotional development are strengthened.

8 A LITERARY EXAMPLE OF MALADAPTIVE RESPONSE TO POSITIVE EMOTIONS AND ITS PSYCHOSOMATIC CONSEQUENCES
Some Thoughts on Anton Chekhov's 'Grisha'

LITERATURE AND MEDICINE

Howard Brody, in his book *Stories of Sickness*, emphasises that doctors can increase their compassion for their patients by reading literature (Brody 1987). He believes that an openness to and acceptance of a story that captures a character's emotional response to an illness or life situation is one of the key ingredients of the compassion we seek. Narrative-based medicine, by paying attention to the stories of patients, aims to equip doctors with the skills to enhance the personal autonomy and self-respect of their patients by increasing their awareness of the richness of their emotional response to life situations. It is within this tradition that I would like to discuss a short story by Anton Chekhov, whose work I always find inspiring.

Anton Chekhov was twenty-six years old and had been a doctor for two years when he wrote this short story in 1886. Like Winnicott, Chekhov had a remarkable ability to enter imaginatively into the life of his subjects and describe in minute detail their feelings and behaviour. I think that this short story is a wonderful illustration of the consequences of failing to recognise, acknowledge and respond adaptively to a toddler's positive emotions of interest and joy in the world he is discovering.

'GRISHA'

Grisha, a chubby little boy born two years and eight months ago, is out for a walk in the park with his nanny. He is wearing a long felt pelisse, a scarf, a big cap with a fur bobble, and warm overshoes. He feels hot and stuffy, and to make matters worse the April sun is shining with cheerful abandon straight into his eyes and making his eyelids smart. Everything about Grisha's ungainly appearance and timid, uncertain steps, expresses extreme bewilderment. Hitherto the only world known to Grisha has been a rectangular one, with his bed in one corner, Nanny's trunk in another, the table in the third and the icon-lamp burning in the fourth. If you look under the bed, you can see a doll with an arm missing, and a drum, and if you look behind the trunk, you can see all sorts of different things: cottonreels, pieces of paper, a box without a lid, and a broken toy clown. Apart from Nanny and Grisha, Mamma and the cat often appear in this world. Mamma looks like the doll, and the cat looks like Papa's fur coat, only the fur coat doesn't have eyes and a tail. From this world, which is called the nursery, a door leads to the space where they eat and drink tea. Here Grisha's highchair stands, and on the wall hangs the clock, whose sole purpose is to swing its pendulum and strike. From the dining room you can go through into a room with red armchairs. There is a dark stain here on the carpet which they still point to, wagging their fingers at Grisha. Beyond this room is another one, which Grisha must not enter, and where Papa is sometimes to be seen – a most mysterious kind of person! Nanny and Mamma are easy to understand: they are there to dress Grisha, to feed him and put him to bed, but what Papa is there for – Grisha has no idea. Then there is another mysterious person; that is Auntie who gave Grisha the drum. Sometimes she's there, sometimes she's not. Where does she disappear to? Grisha has looked several times under the bed, behind the trunk and under the settee, but she was never there ...

In this new world, though, where the sun hurts your eyes, there are so many Papas, Mammas and Aunties that you don't know which one to run up to. But the oddest, funniest things of all are the horses. Grisha looks at the way their legs move and is completely baffled. He looks at Nanny to see if she is going to explain it for him, but Nanny says nothing.

Suddenly he hears a terrible tramping sound ... A crowd of soldiers is bearing straight down upon him, marching in step through the park. Their faces are red from the steam baths and under their arms they are carrying bundles of birch twigs. Grisha turns cold with horror and looks enquiringly at Nanny to see if they are dangerous. But Nanny doesn't run away or burst into tears, so they can't be dangerous after all. Grisha watches the soldiers go past and starts marching along in time with them.

Two big cats with pointed faces dash across the path, their tongues lolling out and their tails curling upwards. Grisha thinks he must start running, too, and hurries after them.

'Hey!', shouts Nanny, grabbing hold of him roughly by the shoulders. 'Where do you think you are going? Just you behave yourself!'

By the path another nanny is sitting with a little tub of oranges on her knees. As he walks past, Grisha quietly helps himself to one.

'What do you think you are up to?', shouts his companion, smacking him on the fingers and snatching away the orange. 'Stupid child!'

Grisha would love to pick up that piece of glass which he now sees lying at his feet and gleaming like the lamp in the corner of the room, but he is afraid of getting another smack on the fingers.

'My humble respects!' – he suddenly hears a loud, deep voice say almost above his ear, and sees a tall man with bright buttons.

Much to Grisha's joy, this man offers Nanny his hand and stands there talking to her. The brilliant light of the sun, the noise of the carriages, the horses, the bright buttons – all this is so astonishingly new and unfrightening that Grisha's whole being fills with delight and he starts chuckling.

'Come on! Come on!', he shouts at the man with the bright buttons, tugging at his coat tails.

'Come on where?', the man asks.

'Come on!', Grisha insists. What he wants to say is that it would be nice to take Papa, Mamma and the cat along with them as well; but his tongue says something completely different.

After a while Nanny leaves the park and takes Grisha into a large courtyard, where there is still snow lying about. The man with the bright buttons follows, too. Carefully they pick their way round the blocks of snow and the puddles, then they go down a dark, dirty staircase and enter a room. It is very smoky inside, there is a strong smell of cooking, and a woman is standing by the stove frying some chops. The cook and Nanny kiss each other, then they and the man sit down on a bench and start talking quietly. Wrapped up in his warm clothes, Grisha begins to feel unbearably hot and stuffy.

'What's all this for?', he thinks as he looks around.

He sees a dark ceiling, an oven-prong with curly horns, and a stove which looks like a black hole ...

'Ma-a-ma', he wails.

'Now stop that!', shouts Nanny. 'You just have to wait!'

The cook places on the table a bottle, three glasses and a pie. The two women and the man with bright buttons clink their glasses and drink several times, and the man keeps embracing first Nanny, then the cook. And then all three of them start singing quietly.

Grisha stretches his hand out towards the pie and he is given a small piece. As he eats it, he watches Nanny drinking ... He feels like a drink, too.

'Me Nanny me', he pleads.

The cook lets him have a sip from her glass. His eyes start, he frowns, coughs and for a long time afterwards waves his arm about, while the cook looks at him and laughs.

Back home again, Grisha starts telling Mamma, the walls and his bed about where he has been today and what he has seen. He talks more with his face and hands than with his tongue. He shows them the sun shining brightly and the horses trotting along, the horrible stove and the cook drinking.

That evening he just can't get to sleep. The soldiers with the birch twigs, the big cats, the horses, the piece of glass, the tub of oranges, the bright buttons – all these are rolled into one and press on his brain. He turns from side to side, babbles away and eventually unable to bear his state of excitement any longer, starts to cry.

'You've got a temperature', says Mamma, placing the palm of her hand on his forehead. 'I wonder how that came about?'

'Stove!', howls Grisha. 'Go away horrid stove!'

'It is probably something he's eaten ...', Mamma decides.

And so Grisha, bursting with impressions of the new life he has just discovered, is given a teaspoonful of castor oil by his Mamma.

SHAME OCCURS WHENEVER DESIRE OUTRUNS FULFILMENT

I can imagine the mother of this thirty-two-month-old toddler bringing him to the surgery the following day, expecting the little boy to be seen urgently without an appointment. She would like the doctor to find out what was wrong with her son because he had not been himself last night, he had a high temperature, he was crying, he would not sleep and he seemed to be in pain.

The doctor would examine the obviously healthy child and, finding nothing medically wrong with him, he would have to choose how to respond to the situation.

The doctor who is aware that there is a connection between hurt feelings and physical symptoms is less likely to overreact by investigating excessively and inappropriately. He is even less likely to add insult to injury by suggesting that the child is malingering and making things up. Rather, he is more likely to respond by showing interest in the child's symptoms, sympathy for his suffering and offering a face-saving explanation such as that he does not find anything seriously wrong but if things get worse to bring the child back.

This type of consultation is very common in our surgeries but, as a rule, time pressure obliges us to ignore the circumstances surrounding the development of the physical symptoms. Most of the time it does not matter because the symptoms are self-limiting, but I do believe that our work with patients becomes impoverished if we are not aware of non-medical explanations for the development of certain physical symptoms.

Chekhov's story therefore gives me the opportunity to reflect on the emotional context within which the little boy's symptoms arose.

It is unusual for patients to come to the doctor when they are in the grip of positive, pleasant emotions unless they are experiencing them so intensely that they can be painfully overstimulating. I can remember only one patient whose headache turned out to be related to his excitement about buying a new car.

Interest is the most elusive of positive emotions because it may not be differentiated from the function it accompanies. For instance, Tomkins observes that the affect of interest or excitement is paradoxically absent from Darwin's catalogue of emotions, probably because his own primary affective investment in perceiving and thinking may well have attenuated his awareness in his own sustained excitement in exploration. This might have led him to misidentify the affect with the function of thinking. Just as one may look with accompanying excitement, so may one think with excitement, yet the affect in each case may not be differentiated from the function it accompanies.

According to Tomkins, the positive emotion of interest is triggered by situations that arouse an optimal increase in the intensity and rate of neural activity. Information capable of providing such a stimulus for the infant may come from such things as a bright object above his cot, the smell of his mother, a new sound in the room. Interest may also be triggered by internal sources of stimulation such as a slight increase in hunger, or an image remembered.

The function of the affect interest-excitement is to make us more interested in whatever is going on. When the proper conditions are met the affect is triggered. It causes biological changes throughout the body and is displayed on the face; this takes on an expression of rapt attention, with the eyebrows lowered and the eyes tracking the object of interest.

The affect interest-excitement feeds on novelty, pursues it and creates it. An excited mood can be sustained when an external situation such as an entertainment provides constant novelty, or some internal source produces new thinking, as in the case of creativity. Anybody who writes, paints, composes, dances or invents will gladly tell you how life can be taken over by the excitement generated. The excitement of creativity can be so alien to our normal life that the ancient Greeks believed that new ideas and the emotionality associated with them were the gift of an external being called the Muse. Today we are more likely to attribute the physical sensations that accompany strong emotions to a virus.

Creativity and curiosity are by-products of excitement. However, we must not only think of the creativity of works of art or of revolutionary new ideas. The quest for new experiences is also a creative quest in the broad sense of the word.

Anton Chekhov describes in a masterful and empathic way the impact on Grisha of new experiences. He does not know whether the new sounds and sights of soldiers marching, carrying bundles of birch twigs is something to be afraid of, or not.

His initial feeling of safety is threatened and as he had had no previous experience of a similar situation, he assesses the danger by looking at Nanny's face which does not display fear and therefore reassures him.

His impulse to follow the cats and dash across the path or pick up the bright oranges, indicates that he is bursting to express his excitement in action. Nanny unfortunately misunderstands his motives and restrains him both times in a rough manner.

Grisha is quick to learn that his attempts to elaborate his interest-excitement provokes Nanny's anger. This in turn blocks the new impulse to pick up an interesting, shiny piece of glass.

There is no doubt that curiosity can kill the cat and unbridled interest needs to be modulated in the interest of safety. However it is worth thinking in some greater detail about how Nanny's anger manages to block the expression of Grisha's interest.

Affect theory allows me to speculate that it is not only Grisha's fear of physical pain when he has his fingers smacked that blocks the impulse to express his interest in action. Tomkins has taught us that when a positive affect is interrupted in the presence of the desire to continue to experience it, shame is activated (Tomkins 1963).

The innate affect of shame, like all other affects does not start out like the emotion of shame that we all understand. It is a biological system by which the organism controls its affective output, so that it will not remain interested or content when it may not be safe to do so. Grisha very soon realises that the elaboration of his interest carries the risk of arousing anger in the Nanny who misunderstands his intentions. Later on when he wants to try the drink the adults enjoy, he is given a sip of the obviously alcoholic drink which chokes him and the adults laugh at the faces he pulls. His desire to drink and eat and join in the enjoyment of the grown ups has been interrupted by the unpleasant sensation of the alcoholic drink and their derisive laughter.

Tomkins has written that shame will occur whenever desire outruns fulfilment. Life is full of impediments to positive affect that cause the acute and the fleeting, as well as the chronic and enduring experiences of shame that so influence our lives and the development of our personalities. What we call hurt feelings is caused by the shame affect and these are always moments when a positive affect has been interrupted by the painful affect of shame. Each of us experiences the shame affect differently because of differences in our memories of past experiences of the shame affect and the way these are coassembled with the shame of the moment.

Tomkins starts his chapter on shame:

If distress is the affect of suffering, shame is the affect of indignity, of defeat, of transgression, of alienation. Though the terror speaks to life and death and distress makes the world a vale of tears, yet shame strikes deepest into the heart of man. While terror and distress hurt, they are wounds inflicted from outside which penetrate the smooth surface of the ego. But shame is felt as an inner torment, a sickness of the soul. It does not matter whether the humiliated one has been shamed by derisive laughter, or whether he mocks himself. In either event he feels himself naked, defeated, lacking in dignity and worth. (Tomkins 1963, p. 118)

Shame is a painful experience. It interrupts affective communication and therefore limits intimacy and empathy. The shame response reduces facial communication. The eyelids are lowered, the head and the upper part of the body droop and the individual stops looking at the other person and particularly his face. Small children often see strangers as a novel stimulus and burn with excitement to study their face. However, faces are more than mere sources of interest: they belong to people, and people differ greatly in how they respond to full, avid investigation. There are rules for the investigation of faces. What starts out as a competent trigger for innate interest is now remembered to be the face of a person who might object to staring, who might get angry; in general, one who might not allow the mutualisation of interest which is so important to friendly human interaction. The very face that had just a moment ago been a stimulus for interest can now prevent further examination of the novel situation or of the individual. Suddenly, perhaps providentially, the shame affect is triggered. Eyes that had only a moment earlier been burning with curiosity, are now averted, the bodily posture of fervent interest abruptly interfered with by the slumped neck and shoulders of shame. Quickly the child withdraws behind the safety of his mother's leg, peeking out from behind the mother, darting a glance now and then, still burning with curiosity but now partially restrained by shame. Active, fully-fledged interest-excitement has not been thwarted completely. It has been reduced, impeded, painfully constrained for a little while. The natural desire to explore what he finds compelling will eventually win but at the cost of experiencing shame.

The shame is so painful that most of us tend to focus on the anger that follows hot on its heels and avoid even naming it. However, great observers of human nature have succeeded in describing the experience.

Jean-Paul Sartre, for example, has described shame as 'an immediate shudder that runs through the person from head to foot without any discursive preparation. A disruption so powerful that it feels like an internal haemorrhage' (Sartre 1948).

Darwin saw this confusion of mind as a basic element in shame. Persons in the grip of shame affect lose their presence of mind and utter inappropriate remarks or burst into tears. They are often much distressed, stammer and make awkward movements or strange grimaces. Shame in its base role acts as an impediment to interest-excitement or enjoyment-joy; it can interfere with anything on earth that we enjoy, from the thrill of scientific discovery to the joy of sex.

Wurmser, a psychoanalyst who studied shame in systematic fashion, emphasises in *The Mask of Shame*, the cognitive content of shame (Wurmser 1994). He discovered that during the moment of shame certain thoughts are likely to occur. Some are near the surface, others become accessible only by paying attention to the world of the unconscious as revealed in dreams and free associations. He found that what one is ashamed of clusters around several issues.

1. I am weak. I am failing in competition.
2. I am dirty. I am messy. I am looked at with disdain and disgust.
3. I am defective. I have shortcomings in my physical and mental make-up.
4. I have lost control over my body functions and my feelings.
5. I am sexually excited about suffering, degradation and distress.
6. Watching and self-exposing are dangerous activities and may be punished.

One of the most important groups within the shame family of emotions consists of the feelings we know as guilt.

Although guilt feels different from shame, it appears that guilt involves shame about action. Usually the action is one that has violated some rule or law or that has caused harm to another person. Guilt seems to involve some degree of fear of retaliation on the part of whoever was wronged by our action, so that we may say that it contains a coassembly of shame and fear.

Had Grisha's mother been with him during the day, and had she been sufficiently attuned to his emotional state, she might have been able to modulate the intensity of his interest in a less traumatic way; for instance, by being understanding and providing him with the right words to talk about his feelings. Although Chekhov was familiar with the emotion of shame, having been subjected to his father's cruelty as a child, in this little story he allows us to draw the conclusion that Grisha's upset was related to the overstimulation of his excessive excitement.

However, Chekhov was not trying to explain anything. His genius consisted in a very fine observation of situations and feelings, and it is his observations that allow one with the help of modern affect theory to come to the conclusion that the little boy's symptoms at the end of the day were probably related to the interruption of his excitement about the world by the insensitive and rough behaviour of his Nanny, who blocked the expression of his interest and joy by activating the competing affects of fear and shame. The image of the black, gaping hole of the stove that so frightened Grisha might be understood as a symbolic representation of the negative emotions activated by Nanny's lack of attunement and understanding. It is tempting to speculate that the tendency to treat the somatic manifestations of emotions with physical remedies, as if they were physical diseases, may promote and encourage the somatisation from which so many of our patients suffer.

9 HELPFUL ATTITUDES

THE HUMANE ATTITUDE

The recent explosion of knowledge in the fields of neurobiology, psychology and genetics has made it no longer helpful to discuss whether or not a particular illness is psychosomatic. It is much more useful to use the term 'psychosomatic attitude' to refer to an approach that pays attention to the emotional context within which physical symptoms arise. Such an approach pays attention to possible interactions of psychological, social and biological factors in all patients, whatever symptoms or disorders they may be suffering. However, interest in the emotions of ill people and understanding these as communication signals is delicate and demanding work and requires the acquisition of a number of skills and helpful attitudes.

Winnicott has pointed out that becoming ill involves dependence. This very fact calls for the attitude of dependability in the doctor. As general practitioners we are expected to be humanely reliable, but this is based on the capacity of the doctor to recognise dependence and the ability to handle the feelings that such a position creates in both patient and doctor. When a person is ill and suffering, fear is only a thought away. Our mental well-being is based in part on the illusion of invulnerability. Any disease, particularly if it is severe, bursts this illusion, attacking the premise that our private world is safe and secure. Suddenly we feel weak, helpless and vulnerable.

In general practice we resonate constantly with the emotional communication of our patients. The more serious the disease, the greater the intensity of the feelings that the patient will communicate. The doctor may be called upon to recognise and handle violent feelings, such as revulsion, despair, the terror of abandonment, the horror of loneliness, humiliated fury or the mortification of shame. Feelings of such intensity may well become intolerable for both doctor and patient. This is probably one of the most stressful aspects of being a general practitioner, and our medical education did not prepare us for the task of managing these emotions. This task depends on the skills of emotional intelligence which will determine to what extent our attitude to the patient will be experienced as humane.

An added difficulty is the relentlessness of the pace of consultations. In sharp contrast to the psychotherapeutic hour which lasts about fifty minutes, a general practitioner on a busy day may have to see twelve patients in one hour. This intensity of demand can arouse distress or anger in the doctor who needs to feel comfortable with his negative emotions if he is to continue making himself reliably available to his patients. He has to keep the intensity of his own feelings low and avoid being invaded by his patients' intense negative feelings which can be paralysing or disorganising.

Winnicott, in 'Hate in the countertransference' (1947), has emphasised that as an analyst working with very demanding, psychotic patients he had to be fully conscious of and able to deal with his own hatred. He was aware that his hatred of the patient was expressed by terminating the consultation at the end of the hour. In general practice where there are six to twelve endings in one hour, the doctor who wants to finish each consultation on time, like Winnicott, has to master his anger and harness it in the service of protecting his boundaries by assertively and politely ending every consultation on time, without giving offence. Very short consultations can be frustrating for patients too, but the general practice setting allows the doctor to invite the patient to come back with a longer appointment if necessary, thereby easing the frustration with the hope of future understanding.

THE EMPATHIC ATTITUDE: FEELING WITH THE PATIENT

In the middle of the twentieth century, Michael and Enid Balint and a group of enthusiastic self selected general practitioners began exploring the emotional difficulties in the relationship between the general practitioner and the patient (Balint 1957).

Their research was to provide medical education with a unique instrument for the teaching and development of emotional skills. This relationship, like any other, has to be built on understanding if it is to succeed. However, unlike any other, the doctor–patient relationship demands a very special kind of understanding of both the doctor's and the patient's feelings.

Of all the skills of emotional intelligence, the ability to understand our own feelings and the feelings of the person we interact with, and to act in a way that shapes these feelings and makes them easier to bear, constitutes the core of the art of handling relationships. This ability to see things from the other person's perspective is a developmental achievement and depends on the capacity for self-control. It depends on our capacity to dampen down our anger, distress and excitement and to restrain the impulse to express our feelings in immediate action by pausing to reflect upon what we are feeling and why. The name for this ability, empathy, was coined at the beginning of the twentieth century by E. B. Titchener, an American psychologist. He considered that empathy stems from a sort of physical imitation of the distress of another, which includes an unconscious imitation of his facial expression, which then evokes the same feelings in ourselves. Titchener sought a different word from sympathy that could be felt for the general plight of another, without sharing the other's feelings. Empathy is possible because emotions are communicable. A person in the throes of an emotion broadcasts it and we observers resonate with his transmission. The contagious quality of the broadcast drags the observer into resonance. Its intensity is decreased to the extent that the broadcaster or the receiver learns to modulate the display of his emotion. This is the physiological basis of empathy; the sharing of emotion that accounts for much of the quality of adult interpersonal relationships. We can observe this in a public auditorium when it is essential to the enjoyment of our entertainment.

Because 90 per cent of an emotional message is non-verbal, the key to the intuition of another's feelings is in the ability to read non-verbal information such as the tone of voice, gesture, facial expressions, and so on. Messages such as anxiety in someone's tone of voice or irritation in the quickness of a gesture are almost always taken in unconsciously and responded to without necessarily being aware that emotional communication has taken place. Tomkins felt that it is from our awareness of the way the skin and muscles of the face have been rearranged or distorted by the affect that strikes us, that enables us to assess what we are feeling. We share the affect just triggered in the other person to the extent that we mimic the operation of the same muscle groups. The source of the affect we imitate purposefully, or the contagion we accept passively, becomes the source of the affect we now experience in ourselves (Tomkins 1962). This is the basis of empathy; the sharing of emotion that contributes so much to the pleasure of social experience.

Although empathy is a vicarious emotion, it is much more than emotional contagion. Empathy builds on emotional self-awareness. The more open we are to our emotions, the more skilled we will be in reading the feelings of others. Empathy is our ability to enter imaginatively and yet accurately into the thoughts, feelings, hopes and fears of another person. The ability to stand in somebody else's shoes and to allow them to do the same to us is a developmental achievement and a sign of health (Winnicott 1988).

The failure to register another's feelings is a major deficit in emotional intelligence and a tragic failing in being human. All rapport, the root of caring, stems from the capacity for empathy. It is precisely the lack of these skills that can cause even the intellectually brightest to founder in their relationships and appear as arrogant, obnoxious or insensitive.

LEARNING EMPATHIC SKILLS

Some doctors have a better developed ability for affective resonance than others. When it is not educated, however, this ability can sometimes be a burden. Although emotional resonance is essential for the enjoyment of an entertainment, it is frequently less than useful to be caught up in the anger or distress of a stranger. Affective resonance is so powerful, so distracting a system of interaction, that infancy is the only period in our lives during which we are allowed free range of affective expression. In every society children are speedily taught how to mute the display of affect so that they do not take over every situation in which they cry or become excited. Just as most or all of the affect we broadcast into our environment must be limited by social and cultural forces, we adults are also obliged to learn a number of skills to help us manage the affect broadcast by others. Our whole concept of ourselves as private individuals is based on the idea that we can be alone, free from the intrusive emotions of others. Adult life requires some balance between privacy and communion. The very idea of maturity is based on the expectation that adults can control themselves. Control of affective expression reduces the amount of affect broadcast into the interpersonal environment. It makes life easier for those around us. Those of us who resonate easily with the affect of our patients have to build a shield for protection from the affective experience of the other person, a mechanism which Donald Nathanson has called the 'empathic wall' (Nathanson 1992). This is a skill, a learned mechanism by which we can tune out of the affective display of others.

One way of building an empathic wall would be by refusing to mimic the facial or bodily display of the affect we see in other people. We might for instance, learn to recognise the feeling of contagion, learn to sense the very moment that another person's affect begins to tickle our affect receptors. We might decide to shift attention to something else and stop the process of resonance. We can block completely the experience of affective resonance by this mechanism of distraction, or we can limit it over carefully graduated levels of connectedness. It is this empathic wall that allows us to maintain our boundaries in the presence of other people when they are experiencing or displaying affect. The empathic wall helps us to preserve the unity of the self. Adults who do not learn how to shield themselves from the emotional lives of others suffer greatly because they fail to develop a secure sense of identity. The skill of the empathic wall which controls the phenomenon of affective resonance is perhaps one of the basic skills upon which a mature sense of empathy can be cultivated. Some fortunate doctors are fairly natural at empathic skills. They perhaps learned from their parents to listen to the ideas, feelings and dilemmas of others. But the rest of us who do not have this advantage must learn if we are to function as humane doctors and not simply as technicians, or 'mechanics of the flesh' as one of my patients put it.

Many doctors have difficulty in this area, probably as the result of traditional medical training that can often be abusive and unempathic. We do not teach empathy by being unempathic to our students, or teach kindness by being abusive. There are doctors who not only lack empathic skills, but who are even unaware of their value. Fortunately, unlike our cognitive intelligence which is in part genetically determined and held by some to be unimproved by education and training, emotional intelligence can continue to improve throughout our lives with the right training.

Platt distinguishes between affectively and cognitively based empathy (Platt 1995). The first is a sort of vicarious arousal, a kind of contagious affect. During contact with the patient the doctor experiences certain feelings and asks himself why he feels that way. He very soon realises that the patient has been feeling the same emotion and that the affect has been communicated from patient to doctor. Once this process is understood by the doctor through an act of reflective self-awareness, contagious affect allows him to act towards the patient with greater understanding. Platt believes that

unfortunately many doctors are not very aware of their own feelings. Most doctors are more cognitively than emotionally aware. They even avoid feelings, their own and those of others. In this case they are more likely to succeed with a cognitive approach to feelings. If they think first that they have to include feelings in their understanding of the interaction with the patient, they will do better than if they depend on catching them from him. (Platt 1995, p. 30)

The acquisition of empathic skills is essential because they facilitate a true understanding and this leads to compassion. In Britain, doctors have limited opportunities for the cultivation of empathic skills. Balint groups (Salinsky and Sackin 2000) and the student psychotherapy scheme pioneered at the department of psychological medicine at University College Hospital London are among the best established examples (Shoenberg 1992).

However, a humane medical attitude that is based on empathy and understanding of the patient's experience of his disease is only a potentiality and has to be protected and defended against a variety of dehumanising influences. The changing culture of medicine itself as it becomes more responsive to the imperatives of business is making such care increasingly difficult. The welfare of the patient is often subordinated to the concept of the patient as an economic unit.

EMOTION COACHING ATTITUDE

In my effort to develop a psychosomatic attitude appropriate to the constraints of the general practice setting one of my inspirations has been Henry Krystal's work. This author has devised several modifications of technique for making psychodynamic psychotherapy more helpful to patients who find it difficult to process their emotional arousal cognitively and are therefore not aware of their feelings (Krystal 1988). He objected to the metaphor of emotional discharge because it implies riddance or evacuation. Emotions are often talked about as if they were substances like semen, blood or faeces which build up inside the body until their pressure becomes explosive. In this vocabulary expressing one's emotions is like letting off steam. Indeed, many patients come to the general practitioner demanding help with getting rid of an unpleasant sensation that may be part of an emotional state. Once we renounce the idea that we can help anybody get rid of their emotions, we are glad to find out that we can be helpful in other ways, such as helping patients to tolerate and manage their emotions better by identifying, naming and differentiating their emotions to obtain maximum information from them. Patients need to be acquainted with their emotions as signals, often unpleasant but manageable and essentially self-limiting; to treat emotions as a valuable part of themselves, as signals conveying information about their relationship to themselves and to others.

This therapeutic activity is comparable to a mother's task of helping her young child to identify, distinguish between and verbalise feelings.

In his book *The Heart of Parenting: How to raise an emotionally intelligent child*, Gottman uses the term 'emotion coaching' to describe the parental attitude that promotes emotional intelligence (Gottman 1997).

Emotional intelligence can be considered to be the opposite of alexithymia, encompassing the cognitive skills required to effectively monitor and self-regulate emotions.

In the course of his research on 100 families with normal children, Gottman identified five steps in the emotion coaching attitude:

Step 1: Being aware of the child's emotions.
Step 2: Recognising the emotions as an opportunity for intimacy and teaching.
Step 3: Listening empathically and validating the child's feelings.
Step 4: Helping the child to verbally label emotions.
Step 5: Setting limits to the child's behaviour while helping him to solve problems.

Although the consultation pace in general practice is relentless, it is possible to adopt an emotion coaching attitude during consultation with every patient who presents with physical symptoms. It can be done very simply, by asking the patient whether his physical symptoms worry him and if they do, what is he afraid may be wrong with him. Asking this question constitutes a thirty-second psychological test, because how the patient handles the answer gives a good idea about his level of emotional awareness and the rigidity of his defences. Some patients do not dare name their fear, whereas others are not afraid but are rather impatient with their symptoms and angry with themselves for feeling ill. Because the fear of the unknown is much worse than a named fear, I think that this approach is helpful to the patient because by inviting him to identify and name his fear, it engages him in a reflective process that may reduce the physiological arousal of his negative emotions and make possible an adaptive assessment of the real problem. It also helps find out what to reassure the patient about. Unless I ask the patient what is he afraid may be wrong with him, I may reassure him about something that never occurred to him but is high up on my list of differential diagnoses. If so, the patient who came to the surgery with one worry risks going away with two. Sometimes all I can do in five minutes is find out what the patient's fear is. Once I know, I can decide whether to reassure him that the result of the examination does not justify his fear, whether it is reasonable to investigate in order to rule out such a possibility, or whether to explore the fear and find out more about where it is coming from. For instance, I may ask a patient who worries that his headaches are caused by a brain tumour whether he knows anybody with such a disease. If he does, I may explore his feelings about that person.

When the patient is given the opportunity to talk about his feelings, he may be able to recognise that some of his physical symptoms can be explained by the physiological arousal of his emotional state which is understood and acknowledged. This recognition may break the cycle of frequent visits to the doctor and frequent requests for investigations.

George Vaillant, in his book *The Wisdom of the Ego*, asked how we learn to master powerful affects. How do we adults learn to say and to appreciate not that we are 'tired' or 'upset' or 'feeling anyhow' but that we are angry or sad or embarrassed or humiliated? Often we learn to do so only by having another person who can hold us empathically and help us to bear and identify our pain (Vaillant 1993).

These ideas are also close to Winnicott's, who, in *Playing and Reality*, emphasised the importance of a playful engagement of the therapist with his patient, which may encourage the patient's own capacity for playing with thoughts, ideas and images, so that he can develop further the symbolic and cognitive elaboration of his affective life (Winnicott 1971b).

However, to engage with a child or an adult patient in emotion coaching requires some degree of patience and creativity. Most importantly, parents and doctors need to be in a reasonably undistracted and calm frame of mind to do well. For this reason it is particularly challenging to adopt this attitude in general practice where the consultation can be frequently interrupted by emergency calls and where patients are very often seen with five-minute appointments or sometimes as emergencies with no appointment at all.

THE HOLDING ATTITUDE

Donald Winnicott was always very concerned to understand fully the part mothers play in the care of their babies so that the young mother can be protected from whatever tends to get between herself and her child. He thought that if the mother is without understanding of the thing she does so well, then she is without means to defend her own position and may only too easily spoil her job by trying to do whatever she is told, or what her own mother did, or what the books instruct. Winnicott observed that one of the natural things mothers do to comfort their babies is to hold them and cuddle them. Out of studying this very close relationship between mother and baby, he developed the concept of 'holding' to describe what is essential for infant care.

At the beginning of life the concept of holding refers not only to the actual physical holding of the baby's body but also to the qualities of concern, reliability and adaptation to the baby's needs that the 'good enough mother' can offer when she is preoccupied with the baby's care. At this early stage it is necessary to think of the baby as an immature being who is all the time on the brink of 'unthinkable anxiety', which is kept at bay by a very important function of the mother: her ability to put herself in the baby's place and to know what the baby needs in the general management of the body and therefore of the person. Love at this stage can only be shown in terms of body care. Infantile trauma gives rise to 'unthinkable anxiety' which, according to Winnicott, has only a few varieties: 'going to pieces', 'falling for ever', 'having no relationship to the body', 'having no orientation'.

Because there is a parallel between medical care and infant care, the doctors who are prepared to study the mother–baby relationship and particularly the concept of holding, can learn a lot about caring for the emotional needs of their patients. According to Winnicott, in infancy when so much development is starting, two processes are fundamental: maturation and dependence.

At first the environment is essential, but gradually it becomes less so. At the beginning the baby has no awareness of being dependent on the mother. His dependency dawns on the child gradually, depending on the good enough mother's capacity to let him down in not too traumatic a fashion.

The environment does not make the baby grow, nor does it determine the direction of growth. The environment, when good enough, facilitates the maturational processes. For this to happen the environmental provision, in an extremely subtle manner, adapts itself to the changing needs arising out of the concept of maturation. Such a subtle adaptation to changing needs can only be given by a person who has for the time being no other preoccupation and who is identified with the infant, so that the infant's needs are met as by a natural process. At this early phase love is expressed in terms of physical care by adaptation and reliability meeting dependence.

There is an analogy between the activities of the ordinary good enough mother who provides a facilitating environment for the development of her baby's maturation and the activities of the good enough doctor who provides a supportive environment for the unfolding of the patient's innate tendency for integration and self-healing. In medical care the concepts of illness and of being ill bring immediate relief because they legitimise dependence. Encounter with an ill person in the professional setting moves the doctor into the position of one who responds to need, with adaptation, concern and reliability. This is a form of holding and it facilitates the healing process which is a regrowing just as much when it concerns the mental self as when it concerns the body. It cannot be artificially hurried.

In later stages of development the concept of holding includes a metaphorical sense of a relationship with a therapist who, by using the right words, gives the patient the feeling that his emotions are understood.

Winnicott felt that a correct and well timed interpretation in an analytic treatment gives a sense of being held physically that is more real than physical holding or nursing. The verbal communication of understanding intimates that the therapist is holding the patient physically in the past, that is to say at the time of the need to be held, when love meant physical care and adaptation (Winnicott 1972).

So holding has a dual meaning. It refers both to the care and handling of the body and to the qualities of concern, reliability and adaptation to need, which are intimately related to the ability to put ourselves in our patient's shoes, to understand empathically his emotions and to find the right words to name them.

THE IMPORTANCE OF THE HOLDING ATTITUDE FOR CLINICAL PRACTICE: FIVE EXAMPLES

Holding the Mother to Hold her Baby

The concept of holding has helped me transform my experience of working in our surgery's baby clinic where, once a week, among other activities, I vaccinate babies. Over the years I observed that several mothers felt guilty about exposing their babies to the pain of an injection, and some appeared overwhelmed by the crying and uncertain about the best way to comfort their baby immediately after the injection. Some would start dressing the child straight away, unwittingly increasing his distress. I even remember one mother who thrust her crying baby into my arms after the injection because she was afraid that he had stopped breathing.

All this is understandable. The natural urge of the mother is to protect her child from pain: exposing the child to the pain of vaccination goes against the grain, although most mothers see the logic of vaccination that the future benefits to the baby far outweigh a little pain now. Donald Winnicott's work inspired my attempt to encourage mothers at the clinic to treat their baby's pain by doing what they naturally do in order to comfort and soothe: cuddle their baby. So just before I give the injection, I ask the mother in an affectionately playful way what she thinks the best painkiller for the pain might be. The mothers are puzzled initially: some mothers say paracetamol; others say the breast, and then they give up. When I tell them that the best painkiller is a good cuddle, they smile with relief. Some say that they were expecting something technical. At this moment I let the mother know that I expect her to give her baby a big cuddle immediately after the vaccination, and as soon as I give the injection I lift the baby from her knees and place it on her chest, so that she can hold the baby and cuddle him tight. I encourage her to get up and walk and rock the baby if she wants to, until the crying stops. Most babies stop crying within a surprisingly short time and I give the mother lavish praise for her ability to comfort her baby so effectively. I stress that she is the baby's best painkiller and she is usually very pleased with the recognition and encouragement of her natural mothering skills.

I believe that this approach constitutes an important lesson for the mother. It takes the emphasis away from her guilt about exposing her child to pain and puts it on her capacity to comfort the baby, which is a very positive contribution and one of her most important natural functions. By encouraging and even directing her, in a friendly and uncritical manner, to hold her infant, a doctor is actually reinforcing her lay belief in what she does best and supporting her in looking after her baby naturally, without feeling ashamed of her understandable protective tendency. The atmosphere in the consulting room becomes intimate and friendly, and such praise of her natural therapeutic capacity, I feel, holds the mother who is holding the baby, so that her holding becomes more effective and confident.

This attitude has transformed a routine activity that any health technician can perform into a unique opportunity to communicate with the mother at an intimate level.

'There is No Such Thing as a Baby'

One day after the evening surgery, a worried mother rang the practice to request a visit for her ill child. On the telephone she said that her ten-day-old baby was suffering from 'projectile' vomiting after every feed and that in between feeds the baby appeared listless. She had to wake him in order to feed him. I was surprised by her use of the word 'projectile', which is used mainly to describe vomiting associated with pyloric stenosis, a medical condition due to hypertrophy and spasm of the muscle fibres surrounding the canal between the stomach and the duodenum. I asked why she used this word. She said that when he vomited, the vomit shot out of the cot! I therefore went to visit her with the possibility of pyloric stenosis prominent in my mind.

I was led to the parental bedroom where the father was sitting on a chair, bottle-feeding his baby. The mother was standing and looking on with a pained expression. I took the opportunity to use the baby's feed as a test for the sign of pyloric stenosis. He looked healthy and was not dehydrated, but as I was talking to the parents I observed that the mother had a towel wrapped around her neck. I asked what had happened. She said that her neck had been painful since the day of the delivery. It happened during labour. She was labouring on all fours and kept turning her head to look at the clock on the wall just behind her. Her labours in the past had always been very fast, lasting about two hours, and the midwife in attendance said that the way she was going she would break her own record! The result was a very painful neck and the pain became worse with every movement. Every time she had to pick up the baby, hold him and feed him the pain became worse and made her wince. The father was also very concerned. 'You are supposed to enjoy the first days with the baby', he said, 'but because of the pain my wife has been very depressed.' By that time I had completed the physical examination of the baby and I knew who the patient was. I explained to the parents that I could not find anything wrong with the baby, but that I felt very strongly that his mother should have urgent physiotherapy to her neck and that I would arrange domiciliary physiotherapy as soon as possible. Then I ventured the suggestion that it was possible that the baby sensed his mother's pain and reacted with one of the limited ways at his disposal. The mother accepted my explanation and seemed pleased with the recognition that her pain was important and needed treatment. I arranged for daily home physiotherapy and kept ringing daily to find out about the progress of mother and baby. By the end of the week the baby had stopped vomiting and the mother was pain-free and very happy.

Donald Winnicott, in a discussion at a scientific meeting of the British Psychoanalytic Society in 1940, astonished his audience by saying, 'There is no such thing as a baby.' This example dramatically emphasises the fact that when we see a baby we also see someone who takes care of the baby. One is in the presence of a nursing couple. Also, this is one of the rare examples in which the factor that destroys the mother's pleasure in nursing the baby is so easily recognised and amenable to simple treatment. This pleasure is very important. Winnicott writes that the pleasure which you can get out of the messy business of infant care happens to be vitally important from the infant's point of view. The baby does not want to be given the correct feed at the correct time so much as to be fed by someone who loves feeding her own baby. The baby takes for granted things like the softness of the clothes and having the bath at the right temperature. What cannot be taken for granted is the mother's pleasure that goes with the clothing and bathing of her own baby. If she is enjoying it all, it is like the sun coming out for the baby. The mother's pleasure has to be there, or else the whole procedure is dead, useless and mechanical. In the present case, the mother's pleasure in holding her baby and her relationship to the baby was spoiled by her painful neck which was interfering with the provision of a good enough environment for the baby. At this stage of development it is necessary to think of the baby not as a person who gets hungry and whose instinctual drives may be met or frustrated, but as an immature being who is on the brink of unthinkable anxiety all the time. Unthinkable anxiety is kept away by this vitally important function of the mother at this stage: her capacity to put herself in the baby's place and to know what this baby needs in the general management of the body, and therefore of the person. Love at this stage can only be shown in terms of body care. When the good enough care in this early stage is disturbed and there is a failure of holding, the baby experiences an interruption of the continuity of his being. The place of being is taken by a reaction to impingement. In this case vomiting and lethargy were such reactions. However, there is a positive aspect to this reaction. The baby's symptoms forced the mother to seek outside help which met her own needs.

One can only speculate about what might have happened to the baby if his symptoms had not been recognised for what they were: a reaction to the failure of holding. Could he have gone on to develop hypertrophic pyloric stenosis? There is some experimental evidence that this might have happened. Graeme Taylor, in *Psychosomatic Medicine and Contemporary Psychoanalysis*, mentions a recent study of hypertrophic pyloric stenosis.

Several investigations have demonstrated a positive correlation between maternal stress during pregnancy, especially in the third trimester and the later development of hypertrophic pyloric stenosis in the infant. As the administration of pentagastrin to pregnant or new-born dogs produces changes resembling pyloric stenosis, Dodge (1970, 1972; Dodge and Karem 1976) suggested that maternal stress leads to the elaboration and transmission of a humoral factor such as gastrin, across the placenta from mother to foetus. However because persistent vomiting does not start until several weeks after birth, Metzner speculated that experiences during the postnatal period might interact with the predisposition proposed by Dodge, to produce the actual lesion. In a retrospective pilot study Metzner (1983) quantified identifiable stress factors in the pregnancies and postnatal experiences of eight mothers whose babies later developed pyloric stenosis. The mothers were not only under stress, but were depressed and experienced a profound sense of incompetence concerning the care of their new-borns. As a result of their emotional unavailability the mothers were not empathically responsive to their babies' styles, rhythms and needs and the usual bonding and reciprocal regulatory interactions were not established. The ever increasing demands of the babies and the difficulty in quieting and soothing them, seemed to intensify the mothers' feelings of inadequacy. It was only after the infants developed vomiting and the mothers were forced to seek outside help that they responded appropriately to their babies' needs. The diagnosis of hypertrophic pyloric stenosis rallied the mothers out of their depressions and they responded to their babies' needs with a new readiness that had not previously been available. As Metzner suggests the symptoms of hypertrophic stenosis seemed to serve the adaptive function of drawing the mothers back into bonding range. (Taylor 1987 p. 166)

Mothers that have it in them to provide good enough care can be enabled to do better by being cared for themselves in a way that acknowledges the essential nature of their task. Initially this task falls on the father, but there are circumstances when help beyond the family circle is needed. When the doctor is able to recognise and meet these needs, he can help re-establish the essential regulatory processes within the mother–infant relationship. Many childhood and adult diseases may be conceptualised as disorders of regulation. The onset of illness sometimes has the adaptive effect of restoring an important interpersonal relationship which is fundamental to psychobiological regulatory functions.

The Man who Could Not Stand on His Own Two Feet
Failure of Internal Holding: Stanley

Stanley was a thirty-year-old messenger in a big firm when I first met him. Ten days after his mother was diagnosed as suffering from carcinoma of the ovary and two days before her operation, he slipped while climbing a ladder at work. As he fell he caught his left foot in a rung of the ladder and his full weight hyperextended his Achilles tendon. He felt acute pain, and after a while his tendon became swollen. Fate was particularly cruel to him because on the day of his mother's operation his flat was broken into and his best guitar was stolen. Before the injury he used to visit his mother every weekend. Since the injury, however, the pain was so severe that he stopped visiting his mother regularly and gave up work.

The background to his mother's illness is important. She had suffered from Irritable Bowel Syndrome for twenty years and had always been terrified that she might have cancer. She had good reason to be frightened, because every female member of her family had died of cancer. She had the impression that in each case, for a long time before the cancer was diagnosed, the general practitioner had reassured the patient that the pains were 'all nerves'. She had had several investigations over the years for abdominal pains which were all negative. One year ago, she presented to the GP registrar, complaining of low, colicky, abdominal pain. He referred her to the gastroenterology department of the local hospital, where she was thoroughly investigated for bowel pathology. During this time I saw her frequently, giving her support. When the investigations were completed, all the results were normal and she was sent home with a supply of antidepressant tablets. Two days later her abdomen became swollen with fluid. An ultrasound scan confirmed carcinoma of the ovary. Her worst fears had been realised, and the doctors, as usual, had made the diagnosis too late. Her husband was very angry and was talking of suing the hospital.

Stanley came to the surgery soon after his injury. He was angry and irritable. He saw our registrar who prescribed analgesic tablets. They did not work and so he returned, complaining bitterly. The registrar was upset by his behaviour and sent him to hospital for physiotherapy. It turned out that he was sent to the wrong department, where they would only treat him if he had sustained a sports injury. After this experience he stayed at home. He wrapped his foot in a scarf and a friend lent him a pair of crutches, but by that time the pain was so bad that he was unable to walk and was confined to his flat. His father had to do the shopping for him as well as look after his ill wife, who by this time had been discharged from hospital and was receiving chemotherapy at regular intervals.

I became involved with Stanley one month after his accident when he made a request for a home visit. When I rang him up he told me that all he wanted was a sick certificate for work. As I was very much involved with the management of his mother's illness at the time, I was interested to find out her son's response to this family tragedy and offered to visit him myself.

He opened the door, hobbling on one foot, supported by crutches. He is a slim man with thinning blonde hair and a pock-marked face with a short beard, but looking younger than his age. He led me into the sitting room where he lived almost in squalor. It was dark, untidy and all the ashtrays were full of cigarette ends. He spoke with some irritability and described his accident and his pain in great detail. 'I can't believe the luck of our family', he said. 'For the last couple of years we cannot stand on our own two feet.' I commented about the fact that his accident happened two days before his mother's operation. He looked at me angrily and said: 'Are you suggesting that my foot is psychosomatic?' I thought that for him this idea would be the ultimate insult and that the patient's trust was at stake at this moment. 'What I am suggesting', I said, 'is that because you felt depressed about your mother's illness, you neglected yourself. Here you are, one month after your accident without any medical help.' He was able to accept this. He said that he had given up going to the surgery because he seemed to upset the doctor he consulted. 'I am sure the doctor can look after himself', I replied. I examined his foot. His Achilles tendon was swollen and tender. I diagnosed post-traumatic tendonitis, gave him anti-inflammatory tablets and organised domiciliary physiotherapy.

I visited him again a week later. He was pleasantly surprised to see me and talked with enthusiasm and at great length about his physiotherapy, and also about the pain in great detail. When I asked him about his mother's illness he answered in the vaguest manner and changed the subject back to his physical pain.

The following week I rang him to find out about his progress and gave him an appointment to come to see me at the surgery in one week. My aim was to encourage him to emerge from the invalid state and move towards independence by offering a regular, weekly therapeutic relationship. At the same time, the home physiotherapy, which satisfied his more dependent needs, was to continue. To my great relief, he attended for the appointment at the right time. After I had listened to a very detailed account of his physical pain, I asked him to describe the change in his mother since her illness. 'When I visited her, she was wearing make up', he said. 'I could not really tell. I made an effort to cheer her up.' Then he looked with a broad smile and asked: 'Why?' He was obviously not ready to talk about painful feelings. After this, he attended every week, on the same day, at the same time; his pain and walking improved and he soon returned to work.

Psychological Care can be Expressed in Terms of Body Care

When I met Stanley one month after his injury and listened to his story, I felt that his condition made sense only in relation to his mother's illness and his family's difficulty in talking about emotions, and that his injury was the result of accident-proneness, which can be the result of depression. I felt that he used physical pain to protect himself from the emotional pain of grief, which must have been much worse. But the most helpful idea for me was that his fall represented a dramatisation of the loss of the internal holding mother, as well as an appeal to the environment to take over the holding function. His first attempt was not successful. The doctor became upset by his anger. His hate had to be met without retaliation and without rejection, unflinchingly. The doctor must survive the patient's hatred. He shared his father's anger about the inability to diagnose his mother's cancer at an early stage. So his pain, which was not improving, served also as a mute reproach to the medical profession for their ineffectualness. After the second visit to the surgery, he withdrew and avoided contact with doctors.

Winnicott has emphasised that it is helpful to think of withdrawal as a condition in which the person concerned holds a regressed part of the self and nurses it at the expense of external relationships. Withdrawal in the absence of a therapeutic person to regress with and to, becomes an illness. The provision of a holding environment alone can transform withdrawal and its sulking into regression. This has a healing quality, since early experiences can be corrected in a regression. There is true restfulness in the experience and acknowledgement of dependence.

Return from regression depends on a regaining of independence. If this is well managed by the therapist, the result is a better state than before the episode. All this depends of course on the existence of a capacity for trust as well as on the therapist's capacity to justify trust. There may be a long preliminary phase of treatment, concerned with the building of confidence (Winnicott 1972).

Stanley's confidence in the medical profession had been shaken. I felt that in the circumstances, to insist on discussing his emotions would be experienced as a refusal to nurse the regressed part of the self. This might force him to become demanding or manipulative, or remain withdrawn. Neglect of his foot injury might also lead to muscle contraction and permanent deformity: a source of future litigation, perhaps.

At this level of regression, psychological care has to be experienced in terms of bodily care. I decided therefore that the most effective way of treating his injury and the accompanying mental state was with domiciliary physiotherapy. Our physiotherapist who, incidentally, had also treated the mother with the painful neck, is a warm, caring woman. She started visiting Stanley three times a week for a combination of massage, ultrasound and stretching exercises: a very intensive treatment. The gadgetry she uses can easily conceal a hidden aspect of the healing power of physiotherapy, the mothering, soothing attention to the body which is of an infantile order and meets the patient's dependency needs.

In parallel, I offered to see him weekly, at the same time and the same day, at the surgery. He found it very difficult to talk about his mother and his feelings about her, and he avoided doing so. At no time did I make an interpretation to him, nor did I force him to look at his emotions. By returning to work his return to independence was complete. This became possible by meeting his dependent needs and allowing him a short period of regression. It was only because he trusted the holding situation that he handed over the nursing of the regressed aspect of the self to the therapists and slipped over into becoming an infant for a little while.

However, his recovery was temporary. In the ten years that passed since the initial episode, his tendonitis has relapsed several times and has been treated in the ordinary way at the physiotherapy department. His condition has interfered with his ability to keep a job for long and the intervals that he spends walking on crutches are increasing. Every time he comes to the surgery for a sick certificate or a disability allowance form, I wonder whether his descent to invalidism could have been prevented had he tolerated his grief, mourned the death of his mother, mastered his feelings and accepted her loss.

Empathic Holding: Brian

Brian was a forty-two-year-old mature, final-year dental student when he came to see me one day with a five-minute appointment. He complained that for three months he had been feeling tired, very tired. His symptoms felt like the flu but without the aches and pains. His concentration had become poor and his stamina had been reduced and all this was affecting his ability to study. Usually he was athletic and liked jogging and playing badminton, but recently he had felt too weak to do any of these activities. However, his sleep was good, his weight steady and his bowels regular.

I asked him whether his symptoms worried him and he said he was afraid that he might be anaemic. This was easy to check and I ordered a battery of blood tests to test for a possible deficiency and asked him to come back in two weeks with a half-hour appointment to discuss the results.

When we met again, I gave him the good news that all the tests were normal. He was rather disappointed that he was not anaemic and he asked me whether he could have a look at his test results to check for himself. I showed him the results and he looked at them in silence for a few moments. He said that he felt weak as if he was lacking in something and if he was anaemic he could have taken some iron to make good the deficit. He was puzzled by the normality of his tests and could not think of an explanation for his symptoms.

I wondered whether his symptoms might have something to do with being a mature student and I asked him to tell me something about his circumstances.

He told me that he was married to a law student who was also in her final year doing her finals and that they have a two-year-old baby girl. In order to give themselves some uninterrupted time they take turns looking after the little girl so that one of them can concentrate entirely on studying. However, the little girl seemed to always seek the attention of the parent who was not available to her and kept interrupting. I asked how he felt about it and he said that he felt frustrated. I asked Brian how he handled his frustration and he said that he usually goes jogging, but recently he did not have the energy to jog any more.

Also, in order to make more time to study over the weekend, he asks some relatives who live in London to look after his daughter for a few hours during the day, but obviously when this arrangement does not fit their own schedule they let him down. If his parents were in London they would have been of much more substantial help. Brian also has a big debt because he had to sell his house at a considerable loss and the bank was breathing down his neck.

Sometimes he has doubts whether he made the right decision to go into dentistry. He is afraid that the way he feels now may stop him from passing his exams and he may find himself in a difficult situation.

I pointed out to him that it sounds as though he is deficient in positive emotions at present. Unlike joy or interest, which are activating emotions giving us the feeling of having a lot of energy, doubt and fear are deactivating emotions. They can make us feel drained and weak. I wondered therefore whether experiencing these emotions could be an explanation for his tiredness. Also I acknowledged that being a dental student is very demanding even when someone is young and has no commitments. In his position he has to make a greater effort in order to succeed.

He looked at me in surprise and was interested to hear this point of view.

'What can I do about it?', he asked.

'The first step is diagnosis', I replied. 'Identifying and naming the emotions you experience is important in order to understand what is going on, so that you can make the necessary adjustments and changes. You have come that far and I am sure that you can complete your studies.'

His eyes lit up and he thanked me for this new perspective on his problem. He asked me to pray for him and I asked him to come and see me again if his symptoms did not improve.

Two years later he has not complained of another episode of tiredness. He passed his finals and is looking for employment.

As Long as You are There to Catch Me When I Fall: Bernadette

Bernadette was a sixty-three-year-old woman who had been registered with our practice for at least ten years. She was a known asthmatic and a heavy smoker and used to come to the surgery with a short five-minute appointment every two weeks for repeat prescription for the diazepam medication on which she was dependent. She wore a woolly hat and large, dark, ski sunglasses that hid her eyes and in which I could see a distorted reflection of myself. She used to come to the surgery with her dog, her only companion, which she left tied outside the waiting room. Usually she complained in a South African accent of various physical symptoms. Over the years I had become used to her style of presenting many physical symptoms using dramatic language in a totally unemotional vocal tone and body language. It was not unusual for her to start the consultation by saying that she was dying because of a nasty cough, a terrible back pain, gasping for breath, and so on. She had had various investigations over the years which had always been normal and usually she was content to leave the consultation with her repeat prescription.

One day, four weeks before Christmas, she came with a five-minute appointment for her usual prescription. She complained by the way that for the last week she had had a headache and double vision when she looked to the right. As I could find no abnormality on a quick examination I thought no more of it.

A week later, however, she came back as always with a five-minute appointment and told me that she had spoken to the out-of-hours general practitioner about her symptoms. He had told her that she needed a brain scan.

I felt annoyed and embarrassed at the implication that I was missing a serious medical condition and asked her to describe the headache.

In her usual exaggerated way she said that she felt red-hot searing pain on the right side of the skull which made her feel sick and shaky and woke her up at night. It was relieved only when she pressed that side of the head.

My face was probably displaying some disbelief because she looked at me reproachfully and said : 'My headache is not psychosomatic you know'.

'So what is your fear then?', I asked

'My fear is cancer in the head and lungs.'

'Why cancer?', I asked. 'Has any of your friends or relatives died of cancer?'

She said that her closest friend, Mary, had a cancerous growth in the head, which was dissolved initially, but then it was found that she had inoperable cancer of the lung. She had died four weeks before Christmas seven years ago. They used to go on holiday together twice a year. Mary's husband, Jonathan, died of a myocardial infarction a week ago, and Mary's daughter-in-law developed a lump on her shoulder and it was found that she had leukaemia. She died three days before Jonathan.

I expressed my shock and said: 'Gosh! Who is going to be next?'

'I think it is going to be me', she said, deadpan.

I asked whether she had been able to cry for these losses but she admitted that she had difficulty crying. She shed all her tears when her brother died of hepatitis B seven years ago.

I had spent more than five minutes with her and was painfully aware of the complexity of the case. On the one hand, I was aware of the theme of grief and identification with her dead friends and relations which had become very strong by the complex confluence of events. On the other, I was aware of this woman's difficulty to express her grief in tears and I knew that 'grief that has no vent in tears makes other organs weep' (see also Chapter 13). I was also aware that a headache that wakes the patient up at night suggests the possibility of a space occupying lesion in the head. As she was a heavy smoker, the possibility of a secondary metastatic deposit in her brain from a carcinoma of the lung was not very remote.

Because general practitioners are not authorised to refer patients for brain scans, I thought that the quickest way of checking the possibility of cancer would be to send her for a chest X-ray. I was hoping that the result would be normal, but to my dismay the X-ray showed a shadow in the right upper zone which could have represented a malignancy.

As soon as I had the result I rang her up to inform her that the chest X-ray showed something abnormal, which could be caused by a chest infection and for which she must take an antibiotic. I also told her that I was making an appointment for her with the chest specialist just in case the X-ray did not clear with the antibiotics.

When she came back to see me five days later she said that the headache had eased and her chest felt clearer, and asked whether the X-ray showed cancer. I had to explain to her that X-rays show only shadows and it is not possible to know for sure without further tests. She said that she wanted to know whether she had cancer before Christmas. 'If I am going to die', she said, 'I will spend all my money, go on a nice holiday and if I see a young man I fancy, I will pay him. Then I will come back and die disgracefully complaining and moaning every inch of the way. I am only 63; I have not lived yet.' 'No;' she contradicted herself and felt confused. 'I have lived. I have done everything I could have hoped to, including getting married three times.'

She saw the specialist a week later. The headache was as bad as ever and as the shadow had not cleared, he arranged a lung and brain scan and he gave her an appointment for Christmas Eve in order to discuss with her the results of the tests.

Four days before this appointment she phoned me at the surgery to complain that she could not move her right eye laterally and when she tried to look to her right she saw eight of everything. I asked her to come to the surgery where I examined her briefly and I confirmed a paralysis of the sixth cranial nerve on the right. She continued to complain of headache and the next day she rang me to say that she could not face going to see the specialist. Could I please phone him and find out the results and then inform her what they were. I asked her what her fear was and she said that she was afraid that if he told her that she had cancer she would breakdown and cry uncontrollably.

I rang the consultant to discuss the results and it turned out that the diagnosis was still far from obvious. Histological examination was essential for the diagnosis and planning of treatment, and the only way to obtain the tissue was to ask the thoracic surgeon to remove the lesion in its entirety because a biopsy through the chest wall would be hazardous. I explained all this to Bernadette over the phone and said that because it was essential for her to meet the consultant, I would come along as well.

'*As long as you are there to catch me when I fall*', she said.

On Christmas Eve we met at the chest clinic and saw the consultant together. The CT brain scan was normal and so we had no explanation for the sixth nerve palsy as yet. She was so relieved to hear that she was not dying of cancer, and that even if she had cancer she could still be cured, that she felt keen to get on with her last-minute Christmas shopping.

When she came to see me in the New Year, without an appointment and one week before her appointment with the neurologist, she was still complaining of a headache. I reminded her that the reason she did not want to go to the appointment with the chest specialist was her fear that she might cry. It was as if she was more afraid of crying than dying. I asked how she would feel if she cried in front of the specialist and she said that she would feel terrible. I wondered whether she meant embarrassed and she thought that the word was an accurate description of her emotional state. I said that it was as though she was afraid she might die of embarrassment. She laughed in recognition of her mortification. I asked her why she was so embarrassed about crying. She told me that she remembered switching off her emotions when she was in her early teens and her parents kept quarrelling between them and using her as a go-between. She felt that neither of them was at all interested in the way she felt and even if she did show emotion, neither would take any notice.

She came for the second time in a week complaining of vomiting and falling about in her flat because she could not see properly on her right side. She had began to find it difficult to look after her dog. Her disability was so distressing that she had cried alone the night before. I asked her whether she felt any better after crying but she had not. It sounded more and more as though she was suffering from a severe brain disease even though the brain CT scan was normal. After discussing her case with the neurologist I prescribed dexamethasone tablets, a drug that reduces brain swelling. A few days later, however, she came back to the surgery to tell me that she could not take the tablets because she was vomiting all the time. She had began to get dehydrated and exhausted and I contacted the neurology consultant to request that he admitted her to hospital. Unfortunately her physical condition continued to deteriorate as more and more cranial nerves became affected and a diagnosis of malignant infiltration of the meninges from a small cell carcinoma of the lungs was finally established. She died in hospital within three months of the onset of her symptoms.

HOLDING INVOLVES A PRECISE UNDERSTANDING OF THE PATIENT'S AND THE DOCTOR'S EMOTIONS

The cases of Brian and Bernadette represent opposite poles of the spectrum of holding. In Brian's case the holding involved an understanding of his physical symptoms in emotional terms. In Bernadette's case, the holding involved my adaptation to her physical needs that were the result of a disease that threatened her survival. Both were made possible by understanding the patient's feelings. Unlike ordinary support, 'holding' depends on a precise understanding of the patient's emotions. This is possible only when the doctor has the capacity to put himself in his patient's shoes and understand imaginatively what the patient feels, can tolerate the patient's emotional state and is prepared to help the patient identify and name his feelings.

The doctor's interest in the patient's emotional state, his respect for it and the accuracy of his understanding may create in the patient the feeling that his fall has been stopped and that his anxiety has been made tolerable.

The present time structure of general practice makes it impossible to extend this type of holding to everybody who needs it. Besides, not everybody wants it.

The consultation with Brian could have ended with giving him the normal results and leaving him alone in his incomprehension. He could have come back then, to me or another doctor, with the same or different symptoms, demanding more and more investigations in order to find medical explanations for his symptoms. However, I wanted to make a positive diagnosis for his tiredness and decided to invite him to come back for a longer consultation to explore the emotional setting within which his symptoms arose. I thought that this would be possible because he was an intelligent man who was not afraid to name his fear. I was also keen to practise with an intelligent man the kind of medicine that takes into account the totality of human nature and does not limit itself to nosology.

Unfortunately we cannot always reassure our patients. Sometimes their worst fears are realised and they develop serious disease. In such cases the emotional context within which physical symptoms arise is complicated by the emotional response to disease. In Bernadette's case, for example, the fact that the clinical and laboratory findings suggested the presence of metastatic carcinoma of the lung did not deny the possibility that some of her symptoms could have been contributed to by the physiological component of the emotions activated by the deaths of her loved ones. In real life we can very rarely, if ever, separate the physical from the psychological. Bernadette's deadpan way of talking about the loss of her friends and the possibility of her own death indicated that she was either not aware of her emotional state or for some reason controlled the adaptive emotional display to the point of seeming indifferent. Although her frequent visits were an indication of her distress and the pattern of her physical symptoms was suggestive of a space-occupying lesion in her head, I wondered whether the headache was also a manifestation of her dissociated grief. She was a lonely person living in a foreign country who was grieving for the loss of her friends and afraid that she, too, might die soon. Understanding her fear and helping her to identify and name it, however, was not enough in her case. A more physical form of holding was needed. Confronted with her physical suffering I had to move, like every doctor does, to a position of one who responds to need with concern, reliability and adaptation. I had to adapt my routine way of working and accommodate her urgent need to consult me without an appointment about her intractable symptoms almost every day, and go with her to meet the chest specialist in order to ensure that she would participate in the management plan rather than withdraw in fear. With her comment, 'As long as you are there to catch me when I fall', she acknowledged my holding function and gave an indication that one of her 'unthinkable anxieties', the fear of falling and of being abandoned, was compounded by the mortification of crying helplessly in front of a stranger. Although she had never cried in front of me, she had said that she would not be embarrassed to do so.

With her physical condition deteriorating, however, there came a time when the holding I could offer her in the general practice setting was not enough to meet her needs and she needed the nursing and physical treatment of inpatient hospital care.

CONCLUSION

In this chapter I discussed some of the emotional skills that are deployed by the general practitioner when his attitude is experienced by his patients as humane. However, it must be emphasised that the physician's ability to respond to his patient's physical and emotional needs with adaptation, concern and reliability and express psychological care in terms of physical care provided in a psychologically informed way, must be complemented by the capacity to protect his own boundaries if he is to survive the relentless demands of general practice.

In the consultation the doctor has to manage at least four variables: the patient's physical symptoms and feelings, as well as his own feelings and time. The doctor who is aware of and can distinguish between his own mood and his emotional responses to the patient's feelings is in a better position to use these as information about his own sensitivities and about the patient's conscious and unconscious motives in trying to provoke certain reactions within the doctor. The precise understanding of his own feelings and the capacity to modulate their intensity and control the impulse to express them in action are among the skills that are necessary to minimise the emotional contagion of his patient's feelings, to preserve his own boundaries and to manage the limited time of the consultation.

In a few special cases, however, a precise understanding of the patient's emotions can provide the experience of having someone who is interested in his feelings, who values them and respects them. This experience amounts to emotional support of a special kind which has been called 'holding' by Winnicott. Holding can give patients the feeling of not being alone in their suffering and that there is someone who will catch them and stop them from falling. This can be a healing experience even for a patient who is terminally ill (Hennezel 1997).

10 THERAPEUTIC PRACTICE

THERAPEUTIC CONSULTATIONS WITH AN ASTHMATIC CHILD PRESENTING WITH PERSISTENT COUGH

My handling of the following case has been inspired by Winnicott's approach to consultations. He has described a method of communicating with children by an exchange of drawings that he called 'squiggles' (Winnicott 1971a). This is a game any two people can play, but usually in social life it quickly ceases to have any meaning. The game can have therapeutic value in the consultation because the therapist uses the material according to his knowledge of what the child would like to communicate and to his theory of emotional development. Winnicott, who emphasised the role of play in all psychotherapeutic contact, did not want this method to be thought of as a technique but simply as one of the many ways of getting into contact with a child on the basis of play. The squiggle game, no less than formal psychotherapy, is performed in the overlap of the therapist's and the patient's area of play (Winnicott 1971b).

The squiggle game is particularly useful in allowing children to communicate safely in an indirect and playful way frightening and dangerous emotions that they could not possibly admit to or that they are not yet aware of. The relief that comes from expressing their emotions playfully and having them accepted and playfully responded to and understood may help in some cases to loosen the knot in their emotional development and encourage a forward movement in the developmental process.

Also in a way analogous to verbalisation, pictorial representation of strong emotions may help to diminish somatic sensations that are associated with their physiological arousal. When I feel that the persistence of a child's symptoms may be related to emotions that have not been understood and responded to adaptively and that the family situation allows for such an approach, I explain to the parent that sometimes giving the child the opportunity to communicate playfully with the doctor may be helpful in providing relief from their symptoms. Therefore I ask both child and parent whether they would be willing to come again with a longer, half-hour appointment, to play the squiggle game. If they are interested I show them what the squiggle game is all about. I put a sheet of plain paper on the corner of my desk between myself and the child and I make a squiggle on the paper and turn it into something recognisable. Then I make another squiggle, and I ask the child to turn it into something with her pencil. Most children's eyes light up at this point and they become eager to play. Although Winnicott felt that this was a method that did not usually require interpretations he did sometimes make them. When I use this method I never tell the child the thoughts I may have about the meaning of the drawings. I show my understanding by what I choose to change the next squiggle into.

Alice: First Contact

Alice was ten years old when I first met her. Her asthma had deteriorated two weeks previously and one of my GP partners had increased her inhaled steroids from twice daily to four times daily. As she had not responded to this measure within a week he had started her on oral steroids and asked her mother, Barbara, to bring her back to the surgery within a week for a review. However, because the medication had not worked, Barbara brought her to the surgery sooner than planned, as an emergency, and I was the first available doctor who could see her. Alice was coughing and choking all the time. Her cough seemed to get worse in the afternoon and persisted all night, keeping everybody at home awake. Because cough rather than breathlessness was her main symptom I felt that referral to the hospital was not necessary. Instead, I examined Alice and reassured her mother that she was doing all the right things and I asked her to bring Alice back in a week's time in order to monitor her progress.

Second Contact

A week later, Barbara brought Alice to the surgery again and told me irritably that Alice was just as bad. She said that the cough was just as violent and that 'she spewed up gunge'. The cough was constant and kept her awake at night. I asked Barbara whether Alice's cough worried her, and she told me that she was afraid in case Alice choked to death, or in case something gave, such as her heart. Then I addressed myself to Alice who was sitting rigidly upright and asked her to tell me in her own words how she felt. In a rasping voice she repeated her mother's words: she was spewing up all this gunge. In her choice of words I observed the strong identification with her mother and in order to elicit a more personal response from her, I asked her in a playful way to tell me about the sleeping arrangements at home and who was disturbed when she coughed. She responded to my playful questioning with amusement. Her mother tried to interfere and answer the questions for Alice but I insisted that I wanted to hear Alice's own words. At this point a glint in Alice's eyes showed me she realised that I recognised her as a person in her own right and valued what she had to say.

I discovered that she was the youngest of three. Her eldest sister Mary was 17 years old and was also an asthma sufferer. Her middle sister Irene was healthy. Because one of the complaints was excessive sputum, I changed her inhaler to one that limits secretions and I asked Barbara to bring her back in a week.

Five days later Barbara requested a home visit for Alice and the doctor who visited ordered a chest X-ray and started her on yet another course of oral steroids.

Third Contact

When they came to see me a week later, I knew that the chest X-ray was normal but Alice's mother said that there was no change in her asthma. I examined her and recorded her PEFR which was 200 with an expected 285 (See chapter 6).

I was rather perplexed by the persistence of the symptoms and I wondered whether the lack of response to medical treatment was due to problems in the relationship between daughter and mother that aroused intolerable emotions. I knew that Barbara was having counselling at the time with our practice counsellor and I decided to discuss Alice's lack of improvement with her.

Breaching the confidentiality of a client is a rare event and is never done without careful consideration. In general practice it is only justified if it is going to help the doctor make sense of the serious physical symptoms of his patient and manage her illness better. From our discussion I learned that Barbara had been seriously abused both physically and sexually by her parents when she was little and by her sexual partners later on. She was going through a very difficult period at the time and she was full of hatred. She found it very difficult to express it and she was afraid that somehow this hatred might damage her children.

Armed with this knowledge I asked Barbara to come and see me on her own in order to explore her concerns about Alice's medical condition.

When we met a week later, she talked again of her fear that Alice might choke to death or that her heart might give. She also told me of her anger and frustration at not being able to help Alice get better. Many times she had been on the verge of taking Alice to Casualty but she stopped herself because she did not want to go over our heads.

I asked what she thought would happen if she did this. Was she afraid that we might retaliate by refusing to see her again?

As a reply she told me the story of her eldest daughter who had a similar episode of persistent coughing when she was one year old. She rang the GP but he took ages to visit. When he finally arrived he was shocked to see how ill Mary was and he immediately sent her to hospital where they diagnosed whooping cough. So by his delay he put her daughter's life at risk.

I assured her that there was no such risk to Alice's life. I did not think she had whooping cough but even if she had she was too old to be at serious risk from it.

The similarity between Barbara's fear that her hatred might somehow damage her children and her fear that Alice's cough might damage her heart reminded me of Hippocrates's observation that the asthmatic must guard against anger. I wondered therefore whether Alice's identification with her mother's anger was interfering with her recovery.

Because none of the pharmacological treatments had worked so far I suggested to Barbara that it might be worth trying a different approach. I told her that sometimes if the doctor gives the child the opportunity to express her feelings playfully by making drawings during the consultation, the physical symptoms become less intense. I suggested therefore that I see Alice for half an hour every week in order to play the squiggle game together. Barbara thought that this was a very good idea. I suspect that her positive response was probably influenced by her own helpful experience of counselling.

First Squiggle Consultation (Drawing A1, see p. 150)

Although Alice had felt well enough to go back to school, her coughing bouts persisted and a week later Barbara brought her to the surgery for our first squiggle consultation.

Her mother wanted to stay in the consulting room and watch, probably out of a mixture of curiosity and mistrust about what I might get up to with her daughter during the half hour. I did not object and so we started our first game of squiggles.

I drew 1 and she added sharp teeth and eyes turning it into a shark's head. *(I was not surprised to see this pictorial representation of oral aggression after all the talk about violent cough, anger and hatred.)*

She made 2 which I turned into a whale by adding a mouth, an eye, a water spout and the sea. She was delighted with my response to the theme of dangerous creatures existing under the surface.

She made 3 which I turned into another fierce creature facing the shark.

Not waiting for my turn she made 4 which she turned into what she called an Ele-polly: a parrot who had an elephant's trunk instead of a beak. *(This enigmatic drawing astonished me. It is a hybrid; a union between two creatures; a parrot and an elephant. It reminded me of the griffin, a mythological composite animal with a lion's body and an eagle's head that had a protective function in ancient Mediterranean lands and features in Lewis Carroll's* Alice in Wonderland. *I was not at all certain about Ele-polly's function though. Was the elephant's trunk an allusion to the trumpeting of her explosive cough, or was there some sexual symbolism?)*

Then she wanted to draw a very small squiggle which I turned into Eeyore, the miserable little donkey from Winnie the Pooh. *(I wondered whether she was trying to represent more accurately her real size. Displays of anger tend to make one appear larger and once anger has been expressed tender feelings have a chance. My decision to change the squiggle into Eeyore was probably influenced by my desire to make sense of her drawing and my belief that behind the anger she was probably feeling sad and frightened.)*

By that time she was very enthusiastic, so when I asked her whether she would like to come again next week to play some more she accepted eagerly.

Two days after this session, the mother requested another home visit. The following day, because she could not stand the cough any longer she took Alice to the hospital at 3 am. There she had yet another chest X-ray and some special swabs to look for the possibility of whooping cough. All investigations proved to be normal. I thought that Barbara had finally found the courage to express her defiance and go over our heads without any catastrophic consequences or retaliation from her general practitioners.

Second Squiggle Consultation (Drawings B2, B3, B4, see pp. 151–3)

Two days after Alice was seen in casualty she came to our appointment and after I looked at her peak flow charts and examined her chest we continued with our squiggle game.

I made 1 which she turned into a little girl by adding hands, hair, nose, eye and legs.

Her 2 I turned into the face of a cheeky child.

My 3 she turned into a map which she divided in two, with a person trapped in each segment. One part was England and the other Ireland.

(I understood this squiggle to represent division, conflict and isolation. The persons trapped in each half of the map are cut off from each other with no means of communicating. I wondered whether the drawing was a representation of a division within herself or between members of her family or both.)

Then she made 4 which I turned into a face.

I made 5. She drew a kite and turned my squiggle into a part of its tail.

She made 6 and its corkscrew configuration suggested the tail of a pig. I added the pig mirroring her previous move by turning it into its tail.

I made 7 which she turned into a face with a long nose.

(I wondered whether the long nose and the kite's tail were some reference to genitals or whether they represented an aspect of the breathing difficulties that she must have had as an asthmatic.)

Then she wanted to play ring-a-ring of roses.

(I felt that our play was about to change into action. I had to encourage her to make a drawing rather than invite us to join her in a dance on the consulting room floor.)

She drew me holding hands with her father who was somewhat smaller than me, then herself as a child, holding hands with her mother who was the same size as Alice and her two sisters. Then between me and her father she drew her grandmother Rosemary, sitting on a swing hanging from her father's hands and mine.

(I think that this drawing represents a remarkable progress from the isolation of the characters trapped in the two segments of the map of Ireland. All the members of her family are now connected to each other by holding hands as they dance ring-a-ring of roses. I am sure she did not know the origins of that dance in medieval England during the black death when it was thought that a ring of roses could offer protection against the plague. Alice has put herself between her father and mother. At first glance it looks as though her face is blank. On closer inspection however one can see that she has drawn herself in profile. Her head is turned left and she

looks at her mother. She has placed her sisters at opposite ends of the drawing as far away from her father as possible. She ran out of space as she was drawing her eldest sister Mary. If size is an indication of importance then I seem to have become at least as important as her father in this arrangement. My position in the drawing seems to reflect her positive feelings for me, a doctor who is prepared to help her look at frightening feelings in a playful way that renders them harmless.)

She took this sheet of paper home with her and brought it back at the next session along with a map of England and Ireland that she had drawn and also some squiggles she had made playing with her sisters.

Third Squiggle Consultation (Drawings C5, C6, C7, see pp. 154–6)

My 1 she turned into a head she called Bart Simpson.
(The Simpsons is a long running TV programme that depicts the adventures of the nation's favourite dysfunctional family. The hair spikes and the teeth reminded me of the jaws of the first squiggle.)

Her 2 I turned into a caterpillar. We talked about caterpillars and then she drew 3, a butterfly.
(The theme of metamorphosis reminded me of her earlier drawing of Ele-polly. I felt that it would probably be precocious of her to be concerned about body changes in puberty and I wondered whether she was alluding to other changes such as the transformation from a quiet peaceful state to one of sexual or aggressive arousal.)

She made 4 which I turned into a figure by adding eyes, an arm and a leg and I made 5 which she turned into Father Christmas.

The mother, who had been present in all consultations, observed everything with great interest and laughed with amusement at each unexpected development.

Then Alice drew 6 which she herself turned into what she called teenage mutant hero turtles!
('Teenage mutant hero turtles' was another favourite TV programme at the time.)

Suddenly we were in a different territory. She wrote the words teenage mutant hero and her mother attempted to correct her spelling. I stopped her, saying that we were not at school now.
(The controlling behaviour of the mother made me think of Minuchin's observation that certain ways in which families relate may encourage somatisation and therefore be responsible for intractable asthma. See chapter 6.)

She went on to draw the weapons of the four main turtles and a whole turtle. She told me that the turtles lived in sewers and had to fight the foot soldiers.

Suddenly we had to be the turtles and be on guard, ready to repulse an attack of the foot soldiers. She switched the lights off and in the darkness we got ready for battle.
(Finally she extended the squiggle game into action. Switching the lights off was a very interesting aspect of our play. Winnicott had often observed that children at times will have the consulting room somewhat darkened. When this happened he

felt that the therapist was within the child playing one role and then another according to her directions.

I felt that the mutant turtles continued the theme of transformation. We were both supposed to be mutant turtles and we had to fight off an invasion of the foot soldiers. Our game was obviously representing some inner battle between strong opposing forces. I was not clear whom the foot soldiers represented but the mutant turtles that live in sewers and fight the foot soldiers conjured up in me associations of anal aggression.)

'I did not know that my daughter was so bloodthirsty' said Barbara laughing.

(Barbara's comment made me aware of another metamorphosis. During our sessions Alice was given the opportunity to express her anger in a playful and symbolic way so that her violent coughing was being transformed into a game about violence.)

Fourth Squiggle Consultation (Drawings D8, D9, see pp. 157, 158)

The following week she came with her father. Her mother had a splitting headache and could not make it. The father was a morose and glum man. He had a night job and so he slept during the day, seeing his children very little. I felt uncomfortable in his presence as he sat rather passively while Alice and I played squiggles.

It was a very tense and lifeless session.

To my 1 she added the head and body of a parrot and an elephant's ear turning it into an Ele-Polly.

(The Ele-polly again!)

She made 2 which I turned into a dog.

She drew 3, one of the shoe people.

I made 4 which she turned into a horse's head.

She made 5 which I turned into a fat girl.

I made 6 which she turned into a kind of face.

She made 7 which I turned into a duck.

She made 8 which I turned into a crocodile.

After this session I felt that perhaps as her GP I had gone as far as I was prepared to go in this psychotherapeutic way. My aim was not to treat the family pathology but rather to help her with the persistent symptoms and as her cough had improved considerably I felt that I had achieved my aim. However Barbara told our counsellor that Alice valued her relationship with me very much and the counsellor urged me to continue seeing her.

Fifth Squiggle Consultation (Drawings E10, E11, E12, E13, E14, see pp. 159–63)

The following week she came again with her father. This proved to be an extraordinary consultation.

Alice asked me whether it would be all right for her father to play with us. The suggestion took me by surprise because I was considering asking him to wait outside. However I decided to let Alice lead and I agreed. We all sat round the corner of my desk and began.

I made 1 which her father turned into a face.

He made 2 which Alice turned into an elephant by extending the trunk and adding the ears the eyes and the tusks. I asked her what she liked about elephants and she told me that an elephant had squirted her once in the zoo! *(I felt that her reply favoured the idea of the trunk as a representation of male genitals rather than as a breathing apparatus.)*

Then she made 3 which I turned into a duck.

She made 4 which her father turned into a cat.

I made 5 which she turned into a boy and girl cuddling, called Molly and Dolly. She put her cheek against her father's cheek to show me what she meant.

(Was this a show of love for her father? And was there any significance in the fact that Ele-polly rhymes with Molly and Dolly?)

Then the father made 6 which I turned into a face smoking a cigarette.

She drew 7 which her father turned into an airplane.

He said that when he was younger he had taken flying lessons.

Then I made 8 which she turned into a cup into which a drink was being poured.

She drew 9 which her father turned into the topsail of a sailing ship.

Then her father made 10 which Alice turned into the letter E and then completed the word HELP!

(I was amazed. Was she in danger? Was she trying to tell me something about her relationship with her father? Who needed help? Did she need help to deal with their relationship? I felt that in her drawings she displayed her love for him but perhaps their relationship was more complicated than I thought at the time.)

'Who needs help?' I asked her.

'You do!'

'Who is threatening me?'

'The foot soldiers!!!!'

We were in turtle territory again. 'Where are the foot soldiers?' I asked.

'They are out there,' she replied.

'How are we going to fight them? There are too many!' I said pretending alarm.

'We are going to put a trip wire in front of the door. They will trip, fall down and break.'

I found a tape measure which could stand for trip wire and gave it to her. 'I need a pin' she said.

'Come on Alice,' I said, 'pretend.'

She pressed one end of the tape measure to the wall and gave the other end to her father to hold. He participated with some amusement. She opened the door a little to spy how many foot soldiers were coming. She asked me to switch off the lights. I did so and we were in relative darkness.

The trap was laid. The foot soldiers tripped and fell and we killed them all.

(This was the end of the session and I was amazed at how this child managed to involve her father in play. A father who was not used to playing with his children, who was mostly absent from his family due to his job and who had physically and sexually abused Barbara, was transformed in the consultation into a playing father.)

I congratulated him for playing with us and for being such a good sport.

Alice's asthma had improved considerably since we started playing the squiggle game. She had stopped coughing and choking and her PEFR had risen to 320 with an expected value of 290. The best measurement ever.

She wanted to continue coming to play squiggles every week. Reluctantly, I agreed to do so for the next few months at least. I was reluctant because of Winnicott's warning that seeing a child regularly may raise the expectation of a more intensive psychotherapeutic relationship, which of course I had no intention of providing.

Follow Up

Unfortunately a few months later her eldest sister accused her father of sexually molesting her and the social services became involved. This led to her family splitting up, so that her father had to leave home and find a place to live by himself.

Nine years later, Alice continues to come to the surgery to see me every month or two. Although we do not play squiggles any more she tells me of the developments in her life at school and at home. She uses her inhalers regularly and she has not had another episode of prolonged cough since we first met. She has never talked about the abusive incident.

Conclusion

When I first met Alice and Barbara I felt that the intractable nature of Alice's cough had probably something to do with problems in her relationship to her mother. In particular her mother's controlling behaviour which reduced Alice's autonomy and privacy and her anger with which Alice identified. As she had not responded to medical treatment I offered to give her the opportunity to communicate some of her feelings in an indirect, safe and playful way through an exchange of drawings. This approach helped improve her physical symptoms that were related to strong emotions, probably by promoting their symbolic and cognitive elaboration and diminishing their physiological arousal.

However when I looked at the squiggles again after I learned about her father's abusive behaviour I saw some of them in a less innocent light.

I wondered for instance whether the Ele-Polly drawing represented the union between her father and a member of her family, possibly herself or whether the Molly and Dolly squiggle indicated a closeness that violated personal boundaries. Although it is easy to be wise in retrospect, there is no doubt that it must have been very difficult for Alice to deal with the menacing emotional climate at home. In our last session when I asked her who needs help, she reversed our roles and I was made to be the one who needed help.

In our game I was made to stand for her and ask for help to repulse the invading foot soldiers who could represent the violent and abusive behaviour of her father.

THERAPEUTIC CONSULTATIONS WITH AN ADULT PRESENTING WITH PANIC ATTACKS

Michael Balint, in his pioneering book *The Doctor, his Patient and the Illness*, observed that the general practitioner has the opportunity of seeing patients in the first phases of becoming ill. In other words, he sees them at the stage when they present with functional symptoms which have not yet become organised into a definite illness (Balint 1957).

One of the most important functions of the general practitioner is his response to the patient's symptoms which can contribute considerably to the form of illness at which the patient will eventually arrive. In the following case history I would like to show how my responses to the patient's symptoms modified his initial ideas about their cause and helped him to understand and accept the emotional background of his difficulties so that he could seek the psychotherapy that was the appropriate treatment.

Simon

One summer I received a request for a home visit from Cornwall. Simon's wife, Dinah, had just arrived in Cornwall with her two children to visit her parents, when her husband, who had stayed in London, rang her up in a panic. He wanted her to come back immediately because he felt he was going to pieces with another one of his attacks.

Dinah had been helping Simon with his emotional storms for a long time, but this time she felt she had had enough. She wanted something done about his attacks and she asked me to visit the following day when she would have arrived back home.

At their home, Dinah led me to the kitchen where the family had just finished lunch. There I met Simon for the first time. He was thirty-five years old, but looked much younger than his age, almost boyish. He was handsome, slim and of average height. He spoke slowly in a hesitant, puzzled, uncomfortable manner. He told me that he had been suffering from panic attacks, episodes of rage and periods of depression for at least fifteen years. His symptoms became worse after the death of his mother six years previously, when his first daughter, Margaret, was six weeks old. He was puzzled by the panic attacks during which he experienced many physical symptoms. He had experimented with drugs in his twenties and was worried that he might have damaged himself then. When he erupted with rage he would shout, slam doors, kick the walls and break things. When he felt low he would isolate himself from his friends, stay at home and drink beer. But it was the fear that he found most difficult to cope with.

It was easier to live with rage than terror, which he found incomprehensible. He was working as a builder at the time and he would be too embarrassed to go to work during these attacks because he did not want his mates to see this side of him. They always joked and poked fun at any sign of weakness, and any discussion about feelings was out of the question. His wife had been very good, always being there to look after him and calm him down when the attacks occurred. She was very worried, however, that he might have some endocrinological disorder because he did have a lot of bizarre physical symptoms during his attacks. She was hoping that I might discover the cause with the right blood tests and fix it with the appropriate medication.

Taking the family history from Simon, I learnt that his father had died four years previously at the age of sixty-nine from emphysema. His mother, Margaret, a lovely lady, had died at the age of sixty-five, six years earlier. He had two older sisters and one younger sister.

'You had another sister who died', his wife interrupted. My ears pricked up. I asked him to tell me a little more about this sister.

She was also called Margaret, like his mother and daughter. She had been killed in a road traffic accident when she was sixteen. Simon was eight years old at the time.

I asked how her death had affected his family and he told me that his father lost his joy in living and started suffering from periods of depression. His mother never recovered from her loss. Now that he had become a parent himself, he found the thought of a policeman coming to tell him that his sixteen-year-old-daughter had been killed in an accident unimaginable. However, he did not think that his present trouble had anything to do with the tragic death of his sister because his symptoms had started much later. But he did miss his mother a lot. In fact, he more than missed her. He needed her. When he used to feel bad he would go to her. She would listen to his troubles, cook his favourite food and tell him that he was OK, and he would feel much happier.

At the end of my visit I told him that I did not think he suffered from an endocrine disorder or the after-effects of drugs. In my estimation his attacks had something to do with unfinished business from the deaths in his family and it might help him to have the opportunity to talk about these issues. As he was against the idea of seeing a psychiatrist, I offered to see him for ten twenty-minute sessions in order to understand the issues a little better. He reluctantly agreed to come every Tuesday evening at the end of the surgery.

Towards Healing a Mental Injury

In the first session he talked about the overwhelming intensity of his feelings, which he found disabling. He could be overwhelmed with fear in a supermarket and have to run out into the open air. Even the thought of being in a closed space, such as an airplane in mid-flight, from which he could not escape when he became overwhelmed, was terrifying. He could not discuss this kind of invisible disability with his workmates. If he had a physical injury like a broken leg, it would have been obvious. I told him that he had suffered a mental injury which, unlike some physical injuries, cannot heal with time. He wanted to know how to heal a mental injury and I said that we would have to examine his frightening feelings together. What is overwhelming for an eight-year-old boy does not have to be so for a grown-up person.

Even though he was afraid to examine his feelings in case what he found was too awful to contemplate and he would become overwhelmed by it, he started coming to see me regularly.

In the sessions he spoke slowly, dispassionately and with some hesitation. Margaret, the sister who was killed, was the middle of the five children. Simon and his younger sister were known as 'the kids'. Margaret was going through her adolescent rebellion. She was involved with a group of mods: was coming home late, in spite of her mother's protest, and was wearing clothes and listening to music that her father disapproved of. His mother used to ask Margaret to look after the kids and Simon felt that he was often a nuisance to her. He remembered that the kids used to wind her up and that she did not have enough authority over them like the elder sisters or their mother, because she was almost one of them. He remembered how glad his sister was that, on the night Margaret was killed, she had given Margaret the money she wanted to borrow and they had therefore parted on a friendly note. But Simon could not remember his last conversation with Margaret. On her last night Margaret went out with her boyfriend, who was driving: as he turned a corner sharply, her door opened and she was thrown out of the car.

Simon was in the kitchen with his mother when his eldest sister came home and announced that Margaret was dead. Her words at first were meaningless. It was only when he saw his mother's face distorted by her grief and crying that he was overwhelmed by a sense of dread. He remembered saying that this was the worst news he had ever had and he felt guilty because he could not express his grief in the way his mother and his sisters did. A few days later, in an essay at school, he wrote that his sister had died. When the teacher – who knew nothing about it – read it, she burst into tears and was very sympathetic. Simon felt embarrassed. He did not want to have an abnormal family. He wanted to be like everybody else. He did not want special attention, and at the same time he felt ashamed because instead of showing his grief he had feelings of self-interest. He wondered why children cry over ice cream yet do not cry when something as serious as this happens. I suggested that perhaps there was nobody available to pay much attention to his grief and help him to bear it.

He remembered that after the accident his mother's attitude towards him changed. He remembered the discipline slackening. His mother stopped putting him to bed at 7 o'clock every evening. He would stay up until 9.30 p.m. and he liked this. She stopped reading stories to him at night. Two years later when they moved house his mother was still grieving. He could hear her crying in the middle of the night and he would feel alarmed. He would run downstairs with his sisters to find out what was wrong and she would say that she had remembered Margaret and felt very sad.

He never talked about Margaret with his mother because it always upset her, and when he saw this, he himself felt upset. He remembered cleaning old cupboards with his mother one day and coming across a little box with Margaret's belongings. As soon as his mother saw it she sighed deeply, saying: 'Oh dear', and she became very melancholic. Simon immediately became overwhelmed by a sense of dread that he could not identify or express in words. He remembered that his mother's grief had lasted a very long time and that enough was enough. He wanted her to get back to normal. Finally his sisters confronted his mother with her withdrawal, but he did not remember whether this had had any effect.

One day he was at home with Dinah. The phone rang and, when she answered it, he watched her face becoming distorted by grief as she said: 'Oh, no.' He felt overwhelmed by a sense of dread and realised immediately that his mother had died.

He did not feel the same when his father died, who also withdrew in a big way after Margaret's death. Simon's father had been a member of a folk club, a jazz appreciation society and a member of the socialist party. The house had always been full of people, and everybody had been lively. After Margaret's death, Simon's father lost his pleasure in life and the house remained quiet and empty.

When Simon was overwhelmed by the intensity of his feelings he experienced physical symptoms which made him fear that he might suffer from an organic disease. He complained of tightness in the chest, light-headedness and tiredness. Physical examination and laboratory investigations had always been normal, and I understood his physical symptoms to be related to the effect of his overwhelming emotions upon his breathing pattern. When he was in the grip of panic or rage his breathing became irregular and upper thoracic and precipitated the multitude of symptoms of hyperventilation syndrome. This I treated by explaining the problem to him and teaching him diaphragmatic breathing.

However, his symptoms kept recurring when his fear overwhelmed him in situations where he felt out of control. A typical example was being stuck in traffic inside the Blackwall Tunnel. He felt overwhelmed by dread. He closed his ears and his eyes and started breathing fast and deep. He became dizzy, his whole body started tingling, his vision became blurred and narrow and he could not concentrate. He kept thinking of all the water and earth above him. I linked his fear with the fear of being dead and buried like his parents and his sister, but he told me that he had also been overwhelmed with fear when a train he was travelling in stopped in the middle of a high bridge. I suggested that this association might have been to the fear of falling, of being dropped, of being abandoned by his mother. He realised that he was afraid of being afraid, and once he got used to the fear he felt better.

Another overwhelming emotion was anger. He was very short-tempered and his temper flared up in situations where he felt that he was not listened to. When he got angry he could not think clearly. He started taking his shirt off and opened the windows. I asked him to give me an example of such a situation and he said that it happened sometimes at union meetings when nobody paid attention to his explanations, or at home when he told his children off for being naughty and they took no notice of him.

I made an interpretation at this point, wondering how frustrated he must have felt when his mother, who had been so attentive to him, became withdrawn and preoccupied with her grief after Margaret's death. I also wondered inwardly about how he would feel when our sessions came to an end and I stopped being his attentive listener.

He could see the connection intellectually but he could not get in touch with his frustration during the consultation. He found it very difficult to make the link between his present trouble and what had happened when he was eight. He felt that the one thing he could not stand was a situation of chaos and confusion. When, for instance, there was shouting at home about who would do the cooking and how the housework was to be shared, he felt overwhelmed and wanted to run away. If only he could tell each one of them what to do, then everything would finish in an orderly fashion. I pointed out that the first time he had mentioned being overwhelmed by his feelings and out of control to me was in connection with hearing the news of his sister's and his mother's deaths. He agreed and became thoughtful.

Since he had started coming to see me he had been spending a lot of time thinking about the past, and that worried him because he did not normally do so. He remembered that when, after Margaret's death, their home had emptied he had turned to his younger sister for company and together they had constructed an imaginary country in which they lived. They had drawn detailed maps with fantastic names of cities and towns and had talked of its inhabitants whom they endowed with life.

We were coming to the end of the agreed ten sessions, but Simon was afraid to go back to work. When I helped him to clarify the nature of his fear, he realised that he was afraid that he might be the cause of a fatal accident. Part of his job was to erect scaffolding and he was afraid that if he had one of his panic attacks he might not be able to secure it safely; somebody could fall and get killed. When I suggested that his fear might be related to his guilt about his sister's death, he realised that he wanted to get to the bottom of his problems. I suggested that psychotherapy would be a way forward. Even though he was still apprehensive about exploring his feelings, he was not against seeing a psychotherapist any more. Our sessions had encouraged him to get in touch with his sisters for the first time and find out about the past. During discussions with them he found out that one had been greatly helped by psychotherapy which she started after attempting suicide. He was also reassured by being told that psychotherapy would not be very much different from our sessions together.

I referred him to the psychotherapy department of the local hospital and was looking forward to concluding our discussion in the tenth session. Interestingly, he missed this. I suspect that this had something to do with his difficulty in tolerating his painful feelings about separation.

MOURNING AND SELF-HEALING

When Simon told me in his rather detached way that so many important members of his family had died in the last few years I wondered how well he coped with all these losses.

Human beings adjust to losses and handle the stress inflicted by life's misfortunes with a process of coping, or self-healing, which is very similar to the process of mourning.

Every catastrophic event, along with the obvious losses of those who die, also contains hidden losses, such as the loss of security and of the ability to maintain denial. Similarly, every stress situation involves loss, even if only the temporary loss of the illusion of invulnerability. Effective mourning involves a working-through of the traumatic situation, leading towards acceptance of the reality of the loss and cognitive mastery of the affects that it evokes. During the mourning certain universal emotions arise, which are known collectively as grief. Horowitz has listed these 'Stress Reaction Patterns' in his book *Introduction to Psychodynamics* (Horowitz 1988), as follows:

1. Fear of repetition of the traumatic event.
2. Shame at one's helplessness.
3. Rage at the cause of the disaster which may be vented on innocent bystanders.
4. Survivor guilt.
5. Fear of identification with the victims.
6. Fear of failure to recover from the disastrous event.

I think that this list should also include sorrow for the loss.

The work and process of mourning is useful in considering all situations in which one deals with stress, or in which one has to accept bad developments. The ideal objective of the mourning process is to integrate perception of the new situation and arrive at a new view of oneself.

When emotions threaten to become unbearable or seem to overwhelm the bereaved person, it is helpful to have a number of temporary strategies and devices that ease the distress for a short while and permit a later return to full and conscious attention to the painful emotions. Freud, in 'Mourning and melancholia', gave a classical description of a manoeuvre that helps to increase tolerance of a painful emotion by ensuring that mourning comes in waves. The mourner periodically distracts himself by denying the loss and flying into fantasy. This temporary denial of reality is a resource that the mourner can use to keep grief within tolerable limits (Freud 1917).

However, for the work of mourning to be effective and lead to acceptance of the loss and adaptation to the new reality, the person's emotions must have become sufficiently verbalised and desomatised and his affect tolerance adequately developed. This depends on whether one has learned that emotions are signals to oneself and are limited in duration, or whether one experiences them as dangerous attacks. To the extent that emotions remain undifferentiated and mostly physical, they cannot be utilised as signals to the self in the specific sense that one recognises sorrow in response to loss. Consequently, they can become overwhelming.

HOW DOES AFFECT TOLERANCE DEVELOP

Affect tolerance begins to develop in infancy when the mother permits her baby to bear increasingly intense affective tension by stepping in and comforting the child before his emotions overwhelm him. Her empathy with the child is her only guide and if she fails to prevent the baby's affect from reaching unbearable intensity and the child becomes overwhelmed, a state of psychic trauma may develop. Only when protected from infantile trauma can the child in latency and adolescence gradually build up the ability to bear affects with increasing comfort and security, because an emotion that was overwhelming at some earlier time is subsequently experienced as dangerous and is avoided with dread.

During latency both parents become active in promoting affect tolerance in their child by teaching the family's way to display affect and by offering themselves as models with whom the child can identify. Children whose parents have difficulty in handling affects also have difficulty in developing adaptive ways of dealing with their own emotions.

Krystal has pointed out that another very subtle way in which parents promote affect tolerance in their children is by making the child feel free to take over the soothing and comforting role of the parents, so that the child can develop his self-caring functions. Krystal discovered that although we all have the inborn potential to calm ourselves and find solace, some patients are prevented from doing so by a block or inhibition of their capacity for self-care (Krystal 1988).

These developments are essential preparations for the major task of adolescence: mourning the loss of infantile attachment to the parents, the loss of childhood representation with the renunciation of the infantile models of the world. If the person cannot grieve for these losses he may become caught up in denial or some form of depressive reaction, based on the discrepancy between an ideal view of the self and self-perception. Impairment in affect tolerance renders the adolescent unable to deal with the increased excitement of burgeoning sexual, social and work-related activities.

Simon's Complaint

From Simon's account I realised that he experienced his emotions as attacks that overwhelmed him and made him feel out of control. A person usually becomes overwhelmed when he concludes that the situation he finds himself in is both unbearable and unmodifiable and he therefore recognises his help-lessness. This recognition promotes a diffusion of one's identity and a dependence on others.

Although it is true that the death of a sister is an irrevocable and unmod-ifiable fact and that no amount of crying can bring her back, the complex emotions that such a tragedy evokes can be modified and made bearable with the right help from friends and family and the accomplishment of mourning.

Had Simon been exposed to infantile trauma, he might have experienced an even more radical difficulty with his emotions. This might have prevented him from having the stable family life and work record that he had had. Even so, the death of his sister in his latency, when parents make more conspicuous efforts to help their children develop affect tolerance, interfered seriously with his ability to handle his emotions. Her death was traumatic on many levels. Not only did he lose a sister, but he also lost the attentive responsiveness of his mother and the liveliness of his father who also became depressed.

He dreaded his mother's interminable grieving, she somehow became unable to help Simon with his own grieving. This must have been at least one of the reasons that made him feel overwhelmed whenever his own grief was activated. Another must have been identification with his workmates who exhibited the typical anti-emotional attitude of British culture, heaping contempt on displays of fear and distress. Feeling ashamed about having an emotion may add to the fear and lead to being caught in a self-perpetuating circular reaction of being afraid of being afraid. This reaction compromised Simon's affect tolerance and interfered with his ability to grieve effectively. If losses are not mourned or resolved, they remain as lifelong yearnings or affective debits to be dealt with at a later time. Nevertheless, it is never too late to improve our affect tolerance. It is a lifelong process, and every event in one's life – even dying – presents a new combination of affects which one can learn to handle with grace.

Affect tolerance is the ability to take attention from the somatic sensations of an affect and direct it on to the meaning of that affect.

In order to tolerate our emotions, we must have the capacity to keep the physical sensations caused by the autonomic activation of an emotion within tolerable levels, so one of the first things I did was to help Simon understand that he was not as helpless as he thought. I explained that a lot of his physical symptoms were precipitated by the way his emotions influenced his breathing pattern, and that he could control this in a way that gave him power over his emotions.

By looking at his emotions with interest, I invited him to talk about them and discover their meaning. As interest began to replace fear and shame, he became curious to find out more; by using verbal language to express his emotions he minimised their somatic components further.

By the end of our sessions, Simon had overcome the fear of his emotions and stopped avoiding his sisters. Through conversations with them, he discovered the devastating effect Margaret's death had had on their lives, and he stopped denying the effect it had had on his. He was ready to consider psychotherapy.

I therefore referred him for long-term psychotherapeutic treatment in the hope that his new found affect tolerance would help him complete the mourning arising from the losses and deprivations he had suffered in childhood.

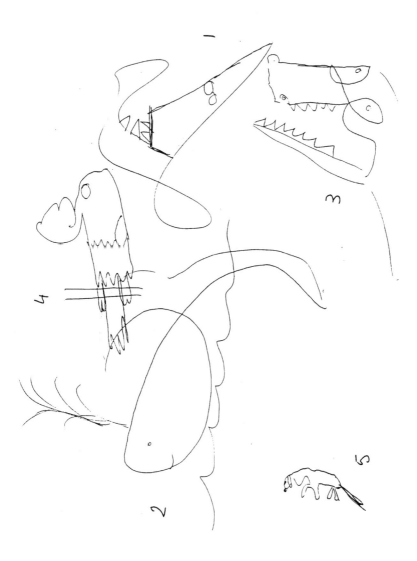

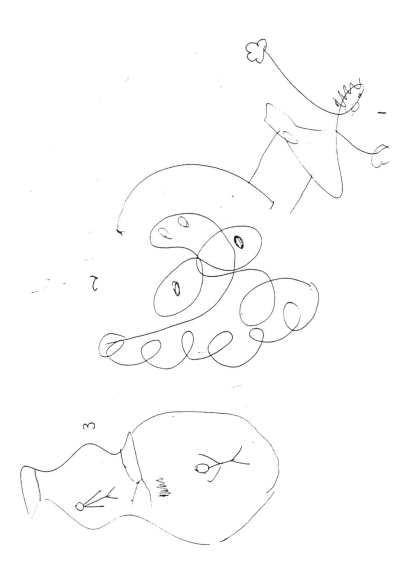

B2

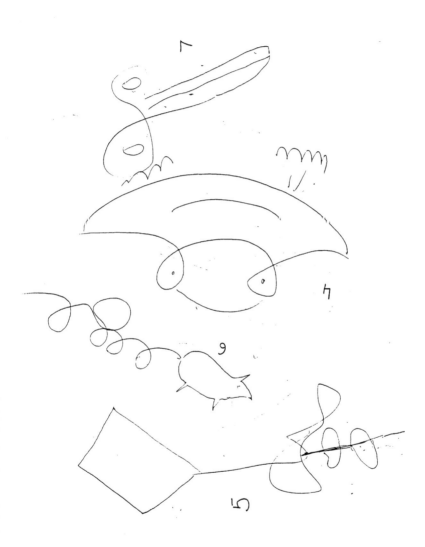

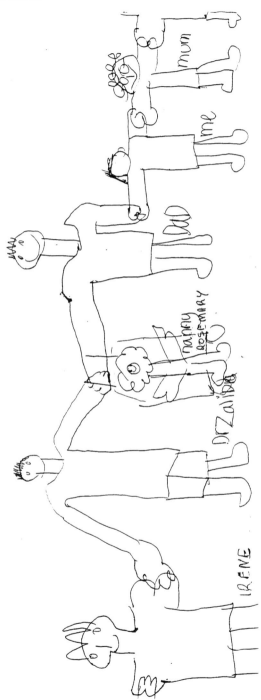

B4

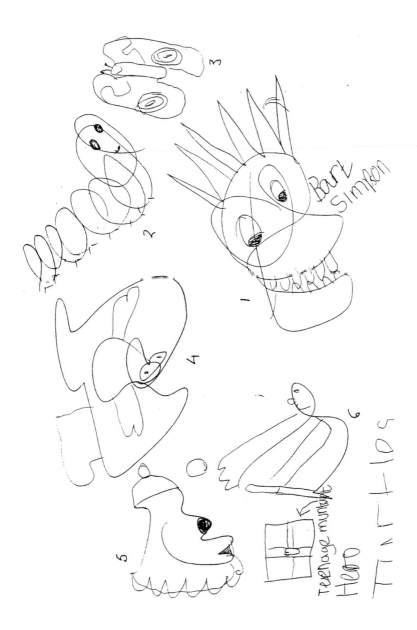

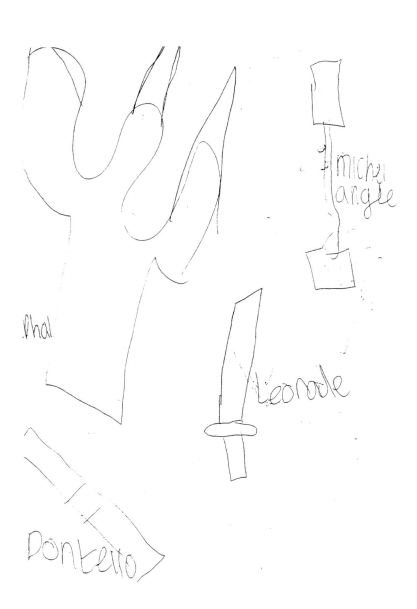

Phal

michel angle

Leonode

Pontetto

C6

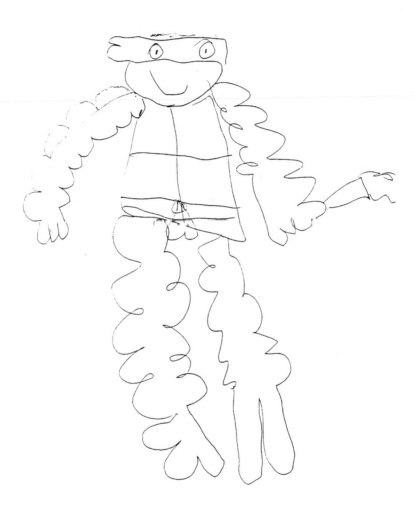

C7

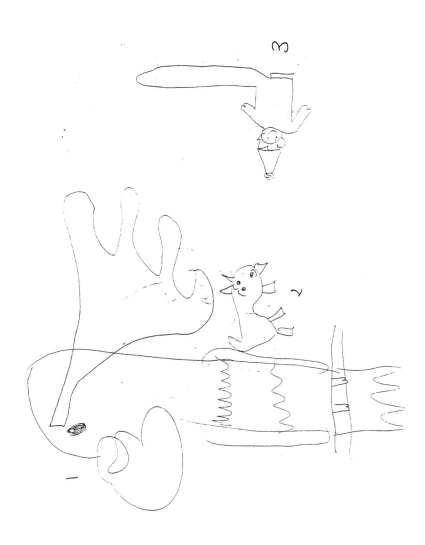

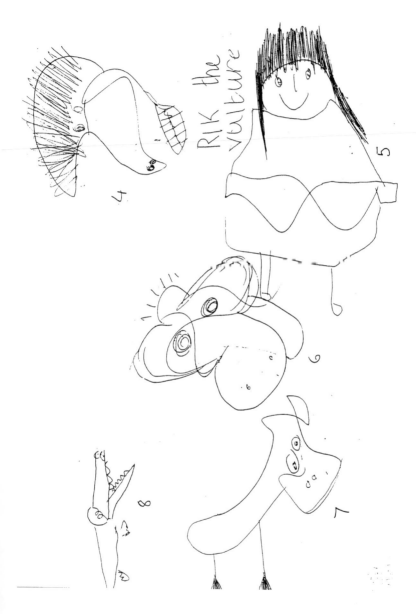

RIK the vulture

4

5

6

7

8

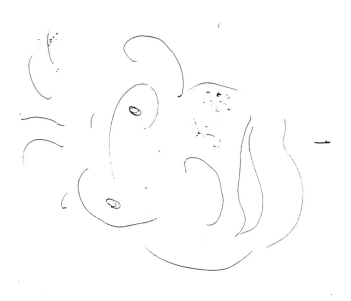

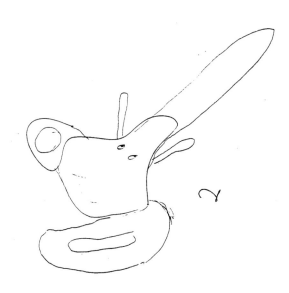

E10

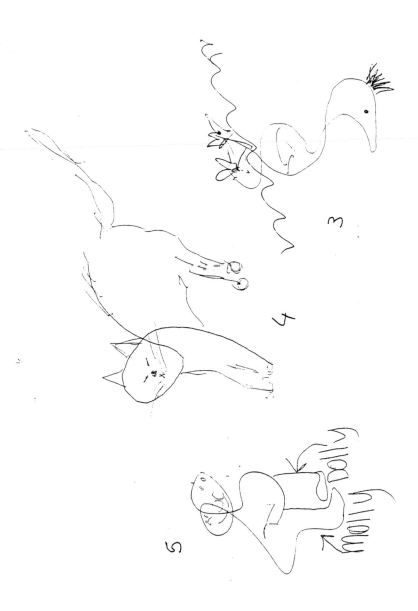

E11

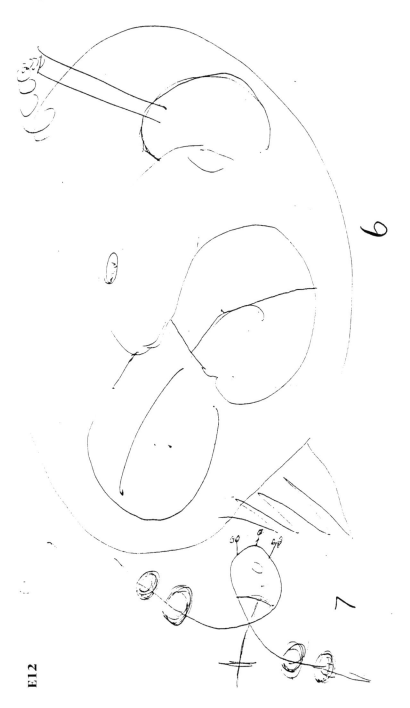

E12

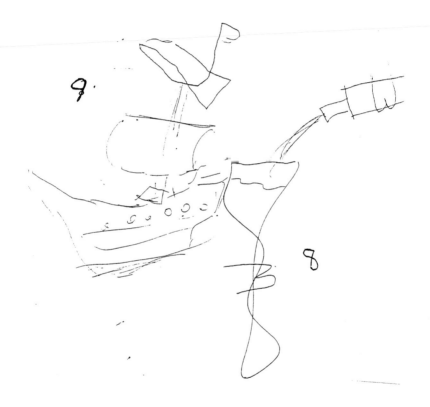

E13

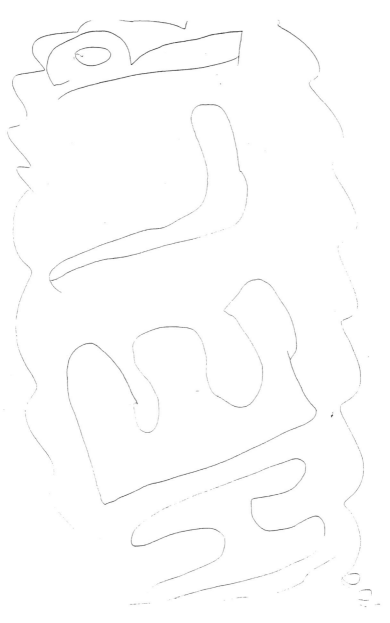

E14

11 OBESITY IS A MULTIFACTORIAL ISSUE

Problems with food and eating are very common in our culture. An eating disorder is probably the commonest symptom with which women in our society express their distress. The idea that misusing food has a psychological meaning was initially explored by psychoanalysts. However, the traditional psychoanalytic view that eating disorders are indications of difficulties with sexuality has been extended by feminist writers. They have suggested that since eating disorders are overwhelmingly a female complaint, the root of the problem lies in the way women see themselves and the pressures they are under in Western culture to achieve a certain shape and size. But what lies behind the distress signalled by eating disorders needs to be explored; it differs from woman to woman.

In most cases the meaning of eating disorders is far from obvious. A modern way of thinking about this is that people *misuse food instead of feeling or understanding something too difficult, or frightening, or unacceptable.*

This something is part of the woman's history, some unfinished business that needs to be dealt with, something unpleasant and painful. Women prefer to misuse food rather than let themselves know about it, but they may pay a very high price for this decision in stunting their emotional development. Eating disorders change the agenda. Something that belongs to the emotional life is being expressed in behaviour. The woman who develops an eating disorder believes that she has found a way of coping with what seems unmanageable. Unfortunately this is an illusion: instead, she creates for herself a much worse problem every time the world becomes frightening by retreating into a compulsive ritual from which she cannot escape (Buckroyd 1994).

Of all the eating disorders, obesity is the most common and it is on the increase in Western culture. In many countries it is classified as a disease and recognised as one of the most important medical and public health problems of our time (Garrow 1988).

The body mass index (BMI: weight in kg/height in m^2) is frequently used as a measure of obesity. Epidemiological surveys have found that between 1980 and 1995 the prevalence of obesity in Britain doubled from 8 per cent to 15 per cent (Wilding 1997).

HELPLESSNESS: THAT SINKING FEELING

The treatment of obesity is often discussed in the media as though it were a simple matter of exercising willpower and sticking to the right diet and exercise programme. Our patients are often misled into thinking that their weight problem can be fixed simply by prescribing the latest slimming tablet. The following case illustrates the complex nature of obesity and the problems one has to face when attempting to treat it.

Betty

I first met Betty when she was twenty-four years old. Her parents brought her to the surgery because for the previous week she had been experiencing chest pains.

As she was grossly obese, weighing over 23 stones (146 kg), they were worried that she had suffered some kind of heart damage. Betty's father worked as a refuse collector and her mother worked in a shoe factory. Betty was the youngest of three children. Her brother and sister had married and left home, but she was still living with her parents.

She had a waddling gait and looked almost as wide as she was tall. She had a round, puffed face with prominent acne, short hair and a rather timid and subdued expression. Her parents wanted me to check her heart and help her lose weight because they were afraid that sooner or later she would develop serious heart disease and die.

I examined her cardiovascular system, but apart from her obesity I could find no abnormality. I sent her to have an electrocardiogram, and before she came back two weeks later for the follow-up appointment I had a look at her medical records.

Ten years earlier she had been referred to the education welfare officer because she was refusing to take part in physical education at school. She weighed 15 stones (95 kg) at the time, and complained that her knees were hurting and sometimes gave way. There were clashes between the school and her parents, and the education welfare officer referred her to the local community physician. He found her to be a perfectly fit young woman who was at risk of becoming depressed and hopeless about her weight. He thought that the only way to start her off with a good weight loss was to admit her to hospital and let the nurses be responsible for her diet. So he referred her to the local paediatrician who found her to be 6 stones above her expected weight and agreed that she needed admission.

She stayed in the local paediatric hospital for three months. She was put on a strict 800-calorie reducing diet and lost 2 stones (13 kg).

Her discharge summary highlights some of the problems that she and her carers faced at the time:

The major problems of her admission were psychological in nature and we relied heavily on the department of family and child psychiatry. Betty absconded from hospital several times. There was talk of suicide, and at one stage she was on regular largactil to tide her over this acute and fairly natural reaction to the prolonged hospital admission and diet. We however weathered these storms reasonably successfully and overall Betty stuck to her diet and we were all very pleased with her continued and steady weight loss. She reached her target weight, looked thinner, was able to wear more attractive clothes and started to take care of her appearance. All this indicated that she could come to terms with her problems and we discharged her on a reducing diet.

However, as soon as she was discharged, Betty regained 3 stones (19 kg) and her weight increased to 19 stones (120.5 kg). She admitted to eating very large meals, and as soon as she had eaten one meal she could repeat it half an hour later. She also nibbled between meals.

Her GP referred her to a consultant physician who did all the relevant investigations and decided to refer her to an oral surgeon for jaw wiring. When she was twenty years old she had her jaws wired and she did very well as far as the weight was concerned, but she developed behavioural problems. She refused to speak and refused to take anything except diabetic orange juice. Because of the danger of starvation the oral surgeons removed the fixation and, needless to say, Betty very quickly put on the little weight she had lost and continued to put on weight thereafter.

Her past history gave little ground for optimism. I spent the next four years trying to find the appropriate treatment for her. By this time Betty was eating almost continuously. Any attempt to restrict her eating would be met with fury. She would shout and sulk and sometimes hit her mother. She would have sweets, cakes, beans on toast for breakfast; a three course meal for lunch; and sandwiches, chips and cheese for supper. She would eat between meals and her family would buy her take-away food in order to keep her quiet. She would drink 4 litres of fizzy drinks per day. She enjoyed food, had no guilt feelings about it and never induced vomiting.

Betty felt that she was addicted to food in the same way a heroin addict is addicted to heroin. If she went for a little time without food she would become irritable and demanding and a member of her family would go out and buy her food or snacks. She became so overweight that she could not reach her feet to wash them; her mother had to wash them for her, resenting this extra demand.

Gradually she stopped going out on her own. She was so uncomfortable in bed that she could only sleep for two to three hours. She did nothing all day except sit in front of the TV feeling bored. One day, four years after we first met, she received a court summons for the theft of £2,000 in catalogue money. She was an agent for the catalogue company, but instead of paying in the money she used it to buy food. Her father understood that there was a vicious circle but felt helpless about changing anything. He told me that Betty's mother wanted her children around her. She went without food when she was little herself and she had sworn not to let the same thing happen to her own children.

Betty started coming to the surgery regularly, expecting me to do something to help her lose weight. I began to dread her visits because in her presence I experienced a profound sense of futility and helplessness. In fact, it was through trying to help Betty that I experienced the meaning of the term 'heart-sink patient' (O'Dowd 1988). It has been suggested that the term describes the physical sensations of the doctor when he experiences the arousal of the parasympathetic component of his autonomic system that accompanies the feeling of helplessness. There is no experience more hateful to a doctor than feeling helpless.

I therefore referred her to the professor of psychiatry at the local teaching hospital who had an interest in the biochemistry of eating disorders. He put her on an appetite suppressant, but her weight continued to increase. He thought that there was no real solution to Betty's problem other than some surgical intervention, and referred her to a consultant surgeon.

The surgeon in question used to treat obesity by creating an ileal bypass, a surgical operation that connects a proximal part of the bowel to a distal part, bypassing a certain length of the bowel which is thus prevented from absorbing nutrients. He had become disappointed, however, with the results of this operation and recommended gastric stapling, a procedure that diminishes the capacity of the stomach, which could only be performed by a specialist at a different teaching hospital.

By that time it had become obvious that the family shared some responsibility for Betty's behaviour, so I referred her to the family therapy department of our local hospital. Unfortunately this proved to be a disaster. Her parents wanted a quiet life and were not prepared to put up with Betty's tantrums when they tried to restrict her food intake.

Two years after our first consultation, I referred her to our local community psychiatrist for a domiciliary assessment. The psychiatrist appreciated the enormity of the problem and put her on Prozac (one of the new antidepressants which is also indicated in eating disorders), and referred her to the professor of human nutrition.

A few days after starting the new drug, Betty took an overdose. She was admitted to the psychiatric ward where she became violent and had to be restrained. She was given Valium intravenously to sedate her. In the ensuing struggle some leaked into the tissues and caused an abscess in the pit of her elbow.

The referral to the professor of nutrition was no more successful. He turned down a request by the community psychiatrist for admission to the metabolic ward for dieting under supervision, on the grounds that such a move would be very expensive. Furthermore, he saw no point in helping Betty lose weight in hospital because when she was discharged no adult would be responsible for restricting the food available to her at home.

The Turning Point

The sense of futility and helplessness was present in every consultation, every two weeks until there was a turning point five years after she first came to see me.

She went to stay with her sister who was very upset because she had discovered that her two children had been sexually abused by her father-in-law. The sister felt very guilty that such a thing had happened under her very eyes and was crying a lot. Betty felt sick and developed severe headache. After three days she had to return home. At the time I thought that the cause of her anxiety was being away from her mother.

The allegations of sexual abuse, however, were serious and the case came to court. Betty when she was twenty-nine years old, came to see me more distressed than usual. She told me that hearing about the sexual abuse of her nieces had brought back memories of her own abuse by her uncle from the age of five to the age of fifteen.

He did everything to Betty seven times a week. He ruined her life. He had died eight years ago, but she kept seeing his face. He had always told her not to tell anybody else because she would never live to see her parents again. When she saw his face in her mind's eye she wondered whether he would come and do the same things to her again. She felt haunted by him. She could see his angry face. She felt that he was angry with her because she talked and was afraid that his spirit might come and separate her from her family. She was afraid to go to sleep at night in case he materialised and did the same things to her.

Betty could not stop herself thinking about him and felt that the only way to stop doing so would be to kill herself. She felt that he had treated her like a prostitute. He abused her from both ends under her parents' noses. He used to ask her to pretend that she was sick and not to go to school and then he would take her to building sites to abuse her, or ask her to accompany him to the betting shop.

She felt guilty for not having spoken out earlier and could not understand why her parents did not protect her.

Her precarious mental state began to deteriorate in front of my very eyes and I referred her urgently to a nurse counsellor in the department of psychotherapy who specialises in cases of sexual abuse.

Two weeks later she started complaining of weakness of the right arm and stiffness of her fingers which she could not relax. A week later she came back to the surgery to tell me that she found the memories unbearable. She wanted to die. As she was talking to me she put her right hand in her pocket, fumbled for a while with her weak hand and pulled out a pair of scissors and with the sharp end started attempting to cut her left wrist in front of my eyes. I was horrified. I demanded that she stop immediately what she was doing and hand the scissors to me. She did so rather reluctantly and then I told her that the weakness of her right arm indicated that a part of her wanted to protect herself from harm.

Although the weakness of her arm was most likely a hysteric conversion reaction, related to the murderous impulses which she had turned against herself and which caused her so much anxiety, the differential diagnosis included organic brain disease, which I could not confidently rule out. I therefore referred her for a neurological opinion in order to share the responsibility which I found overwhelming. In due course she had a brain scan which was normal; and her weakness resolved after the end of the court case that had stirred up her violent feelings.

Two months later she started seeing the counsellor but continued to come and see me. She told me how much she hated her parents but could not tell them this because she was afraid that if they realised that she blamed them for what had happened to her they would kick her out of the house. She felt that she could not survive without them. She felt that when she cut herself or when she contemplated suicide it was her mother whom she wanted to hurt indirectly. Her ideas of violence and the threat of retaliation reached a peak the week before the court case. She was expecting trouble because her family were convinced that the grandfather was guilty, and his own family were convinced that he was innocent. If he was convicted and sent to prison, she would expect his family to attack her family. They were known to be violent. The grandfather's middle son had slashed the face of a taxi driver with a knife and they were capable of burning Betty's family out of their home if her family did not get to them first. However, if the man was found to be innocent and allowed to walk free, then someone from her family – she was not allowed to say who – would have taken something to court to stab the grandfather.

Betty's mother had said that she would back her husband to pursue the man and make him suffer slowly for the rest of his life.

As it happened, there was not enough evidence to convict the grandfather, much to Betty's family's disappointment. I learnt later from Betty's father that he had asked his friends to ambush him and give him a good hiding. So he felt that justice had been done.

Eight years later Betty complained of abdominal pains and went on to say that she wanted to hurt somebody. She wanted to get nasty and violent. I told her that having ideas like these does not mean that she has to translate them into action.

A month later she said that she was afraid to lose weight. Being fat, she was not attractive, and therefore she was safe from male sexual attention. I wondered whether in this way she was also protecting herself from her own sexual arousal.

By that time her weight had stopped being the target of the treatment. The disclosure of sexual abuse drew attention to the pathological family interaction and helped for the first time to mobilise the whole psychiatric team: the consultant psychiatrist, the community psychiatric nurses, the psychotherapist, the psychiatric ward where Betty is admitted from time to time, the family therapy department, and of course me, the general practitioner. Her treatment is going to be long and the outcome is uncertain. Because there are so many people involved we have multidisciplinary case conferences every three months in order to monitor progress and make sure we have a common policy.

In one of our latest sessions Betty gave me a suicide note to read. We discussed her anger with her parents who do not allow her any privacy and read all her mail, and her fear at the thought of leaving home and attempting to live on her own.

I thought that handing me the note was an improvement on her previous attempt to slash her wrists in my presence. She had started to use language to express her feelings. This supported progression from sensorimotor intelligence to early symbolic activity as a substitute for motor behaviour and therefore towards symbolic manipulation of affect, a prerequisite for emotional tolerance.

PSYCHOGENIC VERSUS PSYCHOSOMATIC DISORDER

Obesity is a very good example of a psychosomatic disorder, caused by the complex interaction of emotional and a number of other factors. It contrasts sharply with the psychogenic symptom of weakness of her right arm, which was obviously a hysteric conversion disorder. This is a syndrome characterised by loss of function that appears to be due to a physical cause, but is actually a manifestation of unconscious psychological conflict. It occurs when unconscious forbidden impulses are aroused which produce severe mental conflict that leads to great anxiety. The mind represses suffering by using the unconscious defence mechanisms of conversion and symbolisation. The conflict is then expressed in variable physical symptoms that often have symbolic meaning, such as weakness or paralysis of a limb, numbness, and less often loss or alteration of special sensations including sight and hearing. Conversion of the mental conflict into a physical symptom results in relief from anxiety. This is the primary gain. A proper physical examination of the disabled part makes it obvious that there is no underlying organic pathology to account for the symptoms. However, the hysterical patient, unlike the psychopathic malingerer, is totally unaware of having mentally contrived to produce the symptom. This was Freud's singular and most significant discovery, namely the concept of a dynamic unconscious which could produce a somatic symptom (Wolff et al. 1990).

In psychosomatic disorder, the symptoms have a physical basis that cannot be taken away by simple psychological approaches as it can so dramatically in hysteria, but requires competent and efficient physical treatment. The effectiveness of this can be maximised if the doctor is aware of the emotional factors that contribute to the illness.

HEALTH CONSEQUENCES OF OBESITY

Betty's parents were justifiably concerned about the effect of obesity on her health. It is known that the consequences of obesity can be both physical and emotional.

Obese persons experience twice as much hypertension, osteoarthritis, diabetes and pulmonary dysfunction. Mortality in the youngest age groups is twelve times greater than for persons of normal weight and they are more vulnerable to some forms of cancer sensitive to sex hormones.

Obese persons are perceived by others to have a physical, mental, emotional or moral impairment. Prejudice against the obese is seen in children as young as six years old. Thin and overweight children alike rate obese children as less likeable than children with gross physical handicaps. Later, obese persons are likely to experience discrimination when applying for admission to college and looking for a job. They are assaulted by terms that imply personal responsibility, such as 'lazy', 'weak', 'indulgent', 'self-destructive'.

So it seems that major weight loss is clearly therapeutic and is likely to be accompanied by improvements in both physical and psychological functioning.

SEVEN FACTORS INFLUENCING THE REGULATION OF BODY WEIGHT

As we discovered in Betty's case, however, obesity is much more than the result of eating too much, and the treatment of this disorder goes beyond the simple prescription to eat less.

The discovery that body weight, like body temperature, is regulated by a central mechanism has changed the understanding of obesity. Several lines of evidence suggest that obesity is not the result of a disturbance in the regulation of body weight but, instead, of an elevation of the set point about which body weight is regulated.

In other words, weight, like temperature, is controlled by a central mechanism analogous to a thermostat. Normally we can eat enough to maintain our weight at the point at which this homoeostat is set. In a comprehensive review, Wadden and Stunkard have pointed out that there are at least seven factors affecting this regulation (Wadden and Stunkard 1989).

1. Social
2. Genetic
3. Neural
4. Adipose tissue development
5. Diet
6. Physical activity
7. Emotional

Social

Obesity is more common among women, but a more striking observation is that it is six times as common among women of lower social class as among those of higher class. The same relationship is found among children. A similar though weaker relationship was found among men. The social class of origin is almost as closely linked to obesity as is the subject's own social class.

Genetic

The ease with which obesity can be produced in animals by selective breeding makes it clear that genetic factors can play a determining role in obesity. Animal models have shown how genetic and environmental factors interact. For instance, breeding an overactivity gene into genetically obese mice prevented the development of obesity by increasing physical activity. Human obesity is more complicated, but all the twin studies of obesity have shown conclusively that obesity can be inherited.

Neural

The idea that the body weight may be regulated in obesity as well as in normal weight individuals is relatively new.

It has long been known that the body weight of animals of normal weight is regulated centrally. Only recently, however, has it become clear that animals suffering from various forms of experimental obesity possess the same capacity to regulate their weight. So in animals at least obesity need not be due to a disorder in the regulation of body weight, but instead may be attributed to an elevation of the level about which regulation occurs: the fixed regulatory point.

In most humans, weight tends to remain roughly constant year after year, despite exchange of vast amounts of energy.

The average male consumes about 1 million calories a year. His body fat stores remain unchanged during this time because he expends an equal number of calories.

An error of no more than 10 per cent in either intake or output would lead to a 15 kg change in body weight within a year. The constancy with which adult body weight is maintained by most persons is remarkable, particularly considering how little conscious attention is paid to this task.

Whereas there are many experimental studies of obesity in animals, human studies are very rare for obvious reasons. A few studies have shown that people of normal weight regulate their weight as animals do, but there are no similar studies of obese persons. The little evidence we have suggests that the obese do not regulate their weight at all. How can this be? How can we explain the phenomenon that obese people seem to be the only organisms that do not regulate their body weight? According to an ingenious explanation proposed by Nisbett, obese people do have the capacity to regulate body weight, but the point about which their weight would be regulated, if only biological pressures existed, is higher than that tolerated by the society in which they live. As a result such people go on reducing diets before this point is reached. They are statistically overweight and biologically underweight. In other words, these people exercise restraint as one aspect of the control of their food intake. Such restrained eaters may show counter-regulation of food intake and eat to excess when their habitual restraint is diminished (Nisbett 1972).

The range of disinhibiters is impressive. The experience of such dysphoric emotions as anxiety or depression, along with alcohol and a high-calorie preload can all contribute to removal of the restraint on eating.

If restraint is a voluntary control of food intake, satiety can be described as an involuntary mechanism of control. We stop eating when we are no longer hungry. There are many theories to explain how the loss of hunger is mediated. The most popular relates to low blood sugar: we feel hungry when our blood sugar is low, and when our blood sugar is restored to normal by eating, we stop being hungry. However, a single factor theory cannot explain the function of satiety, because satiety may occur so soon after the beginning of a meal that only a small proportion of the total calorie content of the meal can have been absorbed.

Another factor contributing to satiety is a full stomach. Filling of the stomach, quite irrespective of the nutritive values of a meal, is the major determinant of satiety in single meal experiments.

Adipose Tissue Development

A key to understanding obesity is provided by our knowledge of the anatomy of fat tissue. Increased body fat in obesity can result from increase either in fat cell size (called hypertrophic) or from increase in fat cell number (called hyperplastic), or both. Persons whose obesity started in adult life suffer from the hypertrophic type, while those whose obesity began in childhood are more likely to suffer from hyperplastic obesity or the combined hypertrophic/hyperplastic type. The apparent reason for this is that fat cell hypertrophy is a major stimulus for fat cell hyperplasia in childhood. These children may have five times as many fat cells as either persons of normal weight or those suffering from pure hypertrophic obesity.

This distinction is useful because fat cell size sets a biological limit to weight reduction. Hyperplastic obese persons experience great difficulty in reducing to normal body weight and tend to regain the weight they have lost. For some, achieving normal weight would mean reducing their fat cells to subnormal size. There is evidence that increased cell size and not increased body fat alone, or increased cell number, is responsible for the malignant sequence of insulin resistance and lipid derangement.

Diet

Adult rats maintained on the so-called supermarket diet, which included chocolate chip cookies, salami, cheese, bananas, marshmallows, milk chocolate, peanut butter, sweetened condensed milk and fat rations, gained 269 per cent more weight than controls on normal diet.

Physical Activity

The problem with dieting is that caloric restriction reduces the basal metabolic rate within a few days from starting to diet. This reduction is one of the greatest obstacles to losing weight. Fortunately evidence suggests that mild to moderate physical activity, of the order of twenty minutes' brisk walking every day, counteracts the fall in metabolic rate induced by dieting.

Emotional Factors

Betty's story illustrated vividly some of the emotional factors involved in the maintenance of obesity and stressed the importance of family interactions.

CONCLUSION

It must have become obvious by now that whether to treat obesity or not is an issue of controversy. At the moment there are arguments for and against treatment.

We know that 90–95 per cent of those who lose weight regain it within several years. The failure of obese people to become or remain thin by normalising their food intake follows logically from studies of the heritability of obesity, the biology of weight regulation and the physiology of energy regulation. Desperate consumers of diets are willing to bear the burden of responsibility for failure of treatment in exchange for continued access to it. The debate has shifted from the universal mandate for a single treatment to the matching of available treatments to the individual depending upon the level of obesity and other factors, such as diet history.

Dieting often has negative effects on psychological functioning and can lead to binge eating and even bulimia nervosa. Dietary treatments are costly and unpleasant, and when they fail they damage self-esteem. We should therefore attempt to treat the patient and not the obesity.

Perhaps one of the highest priorities should be to protect people from blame for their condition and have regard to the enormous costs resulting from prejudice against fat.

It has been estimated that obese people lose about £5,000 a year in earnings, spend fewer years in education and that the female obese have a reduced chance of marriage.

The failure of dieting demands a culprit. Either the treatment is not working or the patient is bad, failing to comply with the appropriate remedy.

I think that knowing how complicated a problem obesity can be should protect both doctors and patients from feeling disappointed and helpless when our simplistic treatments do not work. Even when patients arrive at a point in their lives when they are prepared to deal with emotional problems more adaptively, the sociobiological roots of obesity may still create an impenetrable barrier to achieving the ideal BMI.

Finally, I think that if patients' overall cardiovascular risk factors are good and if their obesity does not cause a problem of self-esteem, it is probably reasonable to leave well alone.

12 'GRIEF THAT HAS NO VENT IN TEARS MAKES OTHER ORGANS WEEP'[*]

INTELLECTUAL UNDERSTANDING

When a patient feels physical pain, common sense tells him that the pain signifies damage of the part of the body where the pain is felt. When the skin is jabbed with a pin, the pain is usually accurately localised and the patient can put his finger exactly on the point of injury. However, the ability to localise pain in the injury region is limited to the skin and does not apply when the source of pain is in deeper tissues. Melzack and Wall, in *The Challenge of Pain*, remind us that visceral pain is often felt in bizarre locations (Melzack and Wall 1996).

Doctors are trained to recognise these patterns of referred pain. They are problems that demand intellectual understanding. For instance, inflammation of the diaphragm produces pain which the patient insists is located in the shoulder. The explanation for this strange referral is that the diaphragm, which separates the chest from the abdomen, originates in embryonic muscle tissue that forms in the fifth cervical segment. This muscle migrates during development from the neck to the chest where it develops into the diaphragm, the main respiratory muscle. During this migration, the muscle carries with it its nerve supply, which also originates from the fifth cervical segment. This is the phrenic nerve which runs down the lower neck and through the entire length of the thorax to innervate the diaphragm. Apart from this special migration, the rest of the fifth cervical segment, like all others, forms local skin and muscle. This area of skin, the dermatome, runs in a band from the midline of the back across the top of the shoulder blade and down the upper arm. For this reason pain triggered by nerve impulses arriving from the phrenic nerve may be mistakenly interpreted as coming from elsewhere in the area of skin supplied by the rest of the segment. In other words, pain is referred to the segment of origin of the nerves. Melzack and Wall quote the remarkable study of Jones (1938), who showed that inflating a balloon at various levels of the digestive system sometimes produced pain felt in the back or even at the site of an earlier abdominal operation.

* H. Maudsley, *The Physiology and Pathology of Mind* (1868).

EMOTIONAL UNDERSTANDING

When the patient experiences physical pain, common sense suggests that only physical examination and physical investigations will find its cause. However, psychosomatic research has demonstrated that emotions have physical components which can be perceived in isolation from the psychological experience and felt as physical sensations in various parts of the body. Unfortunately, our ability to think about emotions is handicapped by the dualistic tradition that permeates our training, according to which body and mind are separate entities that may meet and interact. But emotions bridge the body–mind divide because they are at the same time physical and mental and can be pleasant or painful. A very brief way of stating this new way of thinking is that emotions are carriers of information about the relationship to others as well as to oneself. This information is carried by certain affective components. The cognitive component leads therapists to pay attention to the meaning of an emotion as well as to the story behind it; the somatic component refers to the muscular activity and body changes caused by autonomic arousal and neuroendocrine activation, and a hedonic component refers to their quality of pleasure or suffering, and gives them their motivating role.

As already mentioned in Chapter 3, having an emotion or an affect does not necessarily involve awareness of it. Because the physiological arousal of an emotion is sometimes confused with an illness or a 'virus', affect theory reserves the word 'feeling' for the subjective experience of an emotion recognised as part of ourselves. We can recognise that we are experiencing a feeling when all three components occur simultaneously. For this to happen we must be capable of adequate reflective self-awareness and sensitive self-observation. Also there must be no blocks causing isolation or dissociation.

At the beginning of life, emotions serve mainly as communications to another person, usually the mother. They are undifferentiated, their somatic component is very strong and they are experienced mainly as physical sensations, images and impulses to action. Gradually, with the development of verbal skills, the precision and effectiveness of words demonstrate language to be the preferred way of handling emotions. Cognitive processing and symbolic elaboration of emotional arousal helps reduce the intensity of the body language. It also helps to distinguish between different emotions and to experience grades of intensity rather than extremes. These developments are necessary for emotions to become more idea-like and a source of information to oneself rather than another person and require a lot of environmental support if they are to be successful.

Getting to grips with these considerations involves emotional understanding which, according to Michael and Enid Balint, is more complicated than purely intellectual understanding (Balint and Balint 1961). Whereas for the solution of a physiological or mathematical problem it is sufficient to understand the external problem and there is seldom any need to understand ourselves as well, emotional understanding presupposes a fairly keen appreciation of what the emotions under observation mean, both to the observed and to the observer.

A CLINICAL EXAMPLE: MR BAKER

Mr Baker, a sixty-year-old retired postman, came to see me in the middle of a busy surgery on 15 December, complaining of pain in the ball of his right foot. He is a known sufferer from ischaemic heart disease, for which he had a coronary angioplasty five years previously. He is short and obese and speaks softly with a fixed, jolly grin that never varies, as if he is wearing a mask.

This was not our first meeting. We had met for the first time two years previously when he had developed shingles after the funeral of a beloved relative, and I remembered vaguely that he had recently suffered some other significant bereavements. I examined his foot and, finding nothing wrong with it, had a general discussion with him about foot care. Just as I thought that we had come to the end of the consultation and had exhausted his problem, he told me, rather timidly, that he had also had a pain ... 'like a strain' ... in the right lower abdominal area for a month. What started as a straightforward consultation was unexpectedly turning into something more complicated.

As my surgery was running late, I suddenly became very time-conscious, and quickly looked through his notes. I saw that ten years previously he had suffered an episode of severe right epididymo-orchitis (an infection of the testicle and the surrounding tissues), for which he was admitted to hospital for vigorous antibiotic treatment. Since then, he had had the pain on and off, and he was afraid that the infection had returned. I examined his abdomen and testicles and as there was no evidence of any abnormality, I told him so. He looked at me in his usual smiling, friendly way and asked, 'But if there is nothing wrong with me, why does it hurt?' My irritability at running late was compounded by a sense of embarrassment for my failure to find a satisfactory explanation for his pain. I felt that his smile seemed rather incongruous with his complaint, and that if I did not want to lose my credibility and the friendliness implied by the smile, I would have to look harder for an explanation. I needed time to read his notes carefully and remind myself of the discussions we had had, but at the same time I wanted to make sure that I was not missing a serious organic disease. I therefore ordered a number of tests and asked him to return in two weeks, when the results would have been back.

All the results were normal but, looking at his records again, I discovered that his brother had died on 15 December five years previously, and his mother on 16 December one year earlier. He had come to the surgery on the double anniversary of his mother's and brother's deaths.

When Mr Baker returned for his second consultation, I gave him the good news that all the tests were normal. He looked at me with his jolly smile and told me that he still had the pain. I contained the irritation that I could not quite explain at the time, and asked him whether he was afraid that the pain might be due to something serious. He admitted that he was afraid that it might be due to cancer. His brother had died a slow and agonising death with cancer. Then I shared my astonishment with him that he had chosen the double anniversary of his mother's and brother's deaths to come to tell me about his pains, and suggested that December must be the gloomiest month for him. He agreed, but immediately became suspicious that I might be considering the anniversary of the deaths to be 'the cause' of his pain and therefore imaginary. He protested that these things did not bother him, and that his pain was real. As he was talking in his usual jolly grin, I noticed that he wiped away a tear as it rolled down his cheek. I realised then that I was on the right track and that this man had great difficulty in dealing with feelings of sadness. I told him that I did not doubt for a moment that he was in pain and that his pain was real, and to reassure him that I was taking his complaint seriously, I asked him to lie on the couch for a fuller physical examination. As there was some tenderness in his right iliac fossa I was able to tell him that although I could find no evidence of cancer, his pain could be due to spasm of the bowel or possibly appendicitis. If the pain got any worse I could ask a surgeon to have a look at him. I asked him to come back to see me a week later with a twenty-minute appointment.

When he returned for his third consultation, he reported that his pain had stopped after drinking a glass of sparkling water over the weekend. I felt impatient with his lack of insight but kept my feelings to myself. Looking through his notes again, I remembered that I had also seen him in the surgery with similar symptoms just a few days before his mother's death a year previously. At this point I felt confident enough in my understanding of his symptoms to tell him that people do develop physical sensations around the anniversary of the death of important people in their life, and wondered whether his pain had something to do with the feelings he might have about the deaths of his mother and brother. He found this idea an unusual one, and assured me that he was an intelligent man and that what he experienced was not beyond the realm of ordinary human emotion.

He also said that he was a practical sort of person who had discussed the possibility of his own death with his son and had made his will. The idea of death did not frighten him, and he was philosophical about life. He considered humanity as a speck of dust in the universe and that he felt richer for having lived. He might be apprehensive about suffering before death but the actual dying did not frighten him. And yet, I suggested, nobody loses a mother without sadness, and I asked him, how had he felt when his mother died? He said that in fact he had felt a sense of relief because she had Alzheimer's disease and could no longer look after herself. She had never wanted to be a burden to her children. 'Perhaps you felt that for you, your mother had already died – before her actual death?', I commented. He agreed that it was sad that she had lost her mind and that she had become a shadow of her former self, but her death was the end of her suffering. He said all this in his usual jolly, smiling, friendly manner, but his eyes had become moist again. He wiped them and apologised for his watering eyes. I commented on his gesture and asked, was he wiping away tears? He admitted that he was indeed doing so. I asked, might they be tears of sadness? He realised that talking about his mother was a sad topic, but he did not feel any sadness. I reminded him that I had seen him wiping his eyes before, and wondered whether his abdominal pain was real, in the same way that his tears were real – a physical manifestation of an emotion that he could not feel. His fixed grin was somewhat reduced by an expression of puzzlement and thought-fulness. We had come to the end of the consultation and I wondered what symptoms he would present with in a year's time.

Postscript

The following year he requested a home visit because he had an episode of chest tightness, sensations of numbness, loss of balance and incoherent speech – one week after the double anniversary. By the time I visited, he was back to normal. We discussed the differential diagnosis, and he told me that his father had died suddenly of a heart attack seventeen years previously at the age of seventy-seven, and as he was afraid that the effect of his coronary angioplasty was wearing out, he requested a referral to the cardiologist. I thought that this was a very reasonable request and complied with his wishes.

TEARS WITHOUT SADNESS

When we put ourselves in our patients' shoes and imagine the kind of feelings they must be experiencing, we make the assumption that everyone will have the same emotion under similar circumstances, and that a named emotion always refers to the exact duplicate of our own. This very adaptive assumption most of the time confirms our common humanity. However, there are exceptions, and when we meet a patient whose emotions appear not to be what we expect the discrepancy between our expectations and what we observe can be a painful experience.

It is well known that painful feelings of grief are reactivated on the anniversary of the death of important people in our lives and that a positive emotional response to the suffering of grief is sympathy. When a patient experiences grief and talks about his sadness he elicits the doctor's sympathetic response. Usually he is comforted when the doctor listens to his suffering sympathetically, acknowledges and validates his feelings, and accepts his crying with patience and compassion. Such good experiences with the doctor, or with friends and family, help the patient along the journey of mourning and acceptance of his grief and coming to terms with his loss.

When I discovered that Mr Baker consulted me about his physical suffering on the double anniversary of the deaths of his mother and brother, I imagined, by putting myself in his shoes, that I would be grieving for the loss of my own beloved relatives. Thus I was expecting to share in his grief. So when he announced with his jolly, fixed grin at the start of his second visit that the pain was still there, I found the incongruity between his smiling face and the verbal account of his pain irritating.

Michael Balint gave useful advice when he pointed out that the solution to the problem of the feelings of the doctor towards the patient is to treat them as an important symptom of the patient's illness, but that on no account should they be acted upon (Balint and Balint 1961). I have trained myself to follow this advice, so I was able to manage to hold on to my painful feeling and treat it as a prompt to reflect upon our emotional communication. By imagining myself in his situation I could experience some of the sadness and distress of a reactivated grief, but Mr Baker's fixed smile denied any emotional communication at this level. I therefore wondered whether my irritability was my response to our lack of mutuality, to his incapacity to experience sadness, or to his rejection of the emotional experience of grief.

If he had felt distressed or sad, my resonance with his sadness would have provided a bridge between us. The recognition and validation of his emotional state would have created an atmosphere in which he could have revealed and recognised himself. In our discussion, I could have expressed my understanding of his predicament in useful words which could have helped him to reveal more of himself. This might have led to a better understanding of himself and constituted a successful mourning experience which would take him a step closer to coming to terms with his losses. If all this had happened, we would have experienced a satisfying closeness that comes from sharing emotion, and I would have felt effective as his doctor. However, confronted with symptoms uncoupled from sadness as an explanation for suffering, and in the absence of a medical diagnosis, I had an initial feeling of impotence against which I reacted with irritability. Perhaps my feeling of impotence reflected his own toward his distress. This incongruity became even more acute towards the end of the second consultation when his eyes filled with tears, an event that he did not recognise as a sign of distress. Henry Maudsley, a nineteenth-century psychiatrist, said that grief that has no vent in tears makes other organs weep (Maudsley 1868). The opportunity to weep in the consultation is usually therapeutic, not only because it allows a full expression of the emotion of distress, but also because it can provide relief from sadness by communicating emotional suffering, eliciting the therapist's sympathetic response and sharing the emotional experience with him. But despite his weeping, Mr Baker's facial expression continued to display the jolly, fixed grin which suggested an absence of sorrow. In other words, he was displaying only one component of the crying response and he seemed to be unaware of the sadness of which it is usually an expression.

THE FATE OF THE CRYING RESPONSE

Silvan Tomkins, the founder of affect theory, reminds us in his seminal work *Affect, Imagery and Consciousness* (Tomkins 1963) that the crying response is the first that the human being makes on being born. It is a response of distress at the excessive level of stimulation to which the neonate is suddenly exposed.

According to Tomkins, the affect of sadness, or distress-anguish as he prefers to call it, is one of the negative innate affects with which we are genetically endowed.

The face of the crying six-week-old baby already displays the full extent of the crying response. The mouth is open, the corners of the lips are pulled down, arching of the eyebrows gives a sad expression to the face, and there is the characteristic wailing sound that leads to engorgement of the blood vessels of the eyes. The spasmodic pressure on the eye surface and the distension of the vessels within the eyes, according to Darwin, reflexly activate the lachrymal glands, and the baby weeps (Darwin 1872).

The general biological function of crying is to communicate to the individual and others that all is not well and to motivate both to find the cause of distress and do something to reduce the crying response. This can be activated by so many distressors that it is a response of general significance. It enables suffering and its communication. It is as important for the individual to be distressed about many aspects of his life which continue to overstimulate him and to communicate this suffering as it is for him to become interested in things that are changing around him.

Although the communication of distress to the mother is primary during infancy because of the baby's helpless dependency, the significance of this communication to the self increases with age. Just as the drive signal of hunger is of value in telling the individual when he is hungry, and when he should stop eating, so the distress cry is critical in telling the individual himself when he is suffering and when he has stopped suffering. The cry not only has information for the self and others about a variety of matters which need relief, but it also motivates the self and others to reduce it. The face is the major display board of emotions and it is from our awareness of the way the skin and muscles of the face have been rearranged or distorted by the set of motor messages generated by the affect that we interpret what we are feeling (Tomkins 1962).

However, adults very rarely display the full extent of the crying response. The adult has learned to cry by transforming the innate cry and interfering with its expression. So what we see in place of the baby's cry for help is a defence against that cry. He can transform the duration of the crying response and its intensity, and he can also divest it of all the grimaces that accompany it. Another transformation is the display of only part of the cry which then carries the burden of communication. Or the adult face can display the cry but without the characteristic wail as he learns to control the vocalisation. He can also employ a substitute cry, in which there is no sound and no facial response but in which the massive set of motor messages which would have been sent to the face and vocal cords are sent to some other set of muscles instead. Thus they provide some expression of the original cry. There is no part of the body which may not be the recipient of the motor impulses that would ordinarily produce the cry accompanying pain. Tomkins found that some individuals report characteristic contractions of the thigh muscles, others of the calf, the scrotum, the shoulder, or even the gut. Indeed, we very often find a patient complaining of symptoms of Irritable Bowel Syndrome in an emotional setting which could well elicit the crying response.

One of the strongest ways of controlling the overt cry of distress is interference with the grimaces of the cry. Inhibitory messages may be sent to the lips, causing the 'stiff upper lip'; or to both upper and lower lips, causing tight lips, designed to keep the mouth closed and prevent the cry. A more general defence is the mask-like frozen face in which the active facial musculature is kept under sufficiently tight control so that all affects, including distress, are interfered with at the site of expression. I think that Mr Baker's jolly, fixed grin was a variant of these techniques of interference with the facial expression of painful affect. In this way, he deprived himself of the crucial feedback of sensory information from the muscles and skin of his face, which is essential for becoming aware of what emotion he was experiencing.

INTOLERANCE OF SADNESS

Sadness is but one component of grief, a complex emotional state that usually follows a bereavement. Grief includes sorrow, anger, fear, shame, guilt, helplessness; any one of these emotions, or all of them, can be intolerable. The extreme defences mentioned already indicate that there are people who cannot tolerate sadness, even in the smallest doses. There is evidence that such people have in the past most often suffered great shame, anger or fear, along with or consequent to sadness, which are thus added to the emotional pain of sadness; or that earlier on in life they were overwhelmed and made to feel helpless by very intense emotions which flooded them. Thus they are left with a lifelong fear that this experience could be repeated and disorganise them; therefore, they have to defend themselves against the awareness of sadness. In other words, intense fear or shame, or even disgust about it, may block the experience of sadness and interfere with the mourning process.

Mr Baker's difficulty in experiencing the painful emotions of grief may also have had something to do with an experience many years before when he was exposed to death in circumstances that aroused overwhelming distress and fear. He had told me of this experience two years previously when I saw him for three consecutive consultations following the development of shingles. It had happened outside a London Underground station during a raid by the Luftwaffe in 1945.

As the aeroplanes were approaching, the sirens began to sound the alarm and the guns opened fire. There were explosions in the sky and shrapnel started falling and pinging on the pavement. Passers-by rushed for shelter. The station was being built at the time, and a large crowd ran towards it and down the steps. It was so crowded that it was difficult to get in. Mr Baker was one of the last, but he did not know that there was a terrible crush, bodies piled on top of each other lower down the steps. Within a few minuted, 130 people had died. The authorities kept the disaster secret during the war in order to preserve national morale, but finally a commemorative plaque was erected in the station. He was nineteen years old at the time, but he helped to bring the bodies to the surface. He gave this account with his usual jolly grin, but when I asked him how he felt about it at the time, he told me that he could not eat for a week after that tragedy.

The role of shame in denying or repressing traumatically intense feelings has been explored by Wurmser, one of the very few psychoanalysts who have written about this most painful of affects. In his view, the mask-like face of the person who is not aware of his emotions reflects a global denial of emotion motivated by shame and is a consequence of early traumatisation by very severe emotional or physical factors (Wurmser 1994). Mr Baker's timid behaviour in consultations provides some evidence of the link between unawareness of emotional distress and shame. His presenting complaint was a pain in the ball of his foot, an area as far removed as possible from the testicle which he was too shy to name but was concerned about. When he became tearful, he felt embarrassed and apologised for his watering eyes as if they were betraying an insufferable exposure of his weakness and lack of control. According to Tomkins this sadness-shame bind occurs in children when they are treated with contempt, rejection or indifference by their parents whenever they cry. Tomkins observed that the experience or threat of shame every time sadness is activated or anticipated constitutes a radical increase in the toxicity of the experience of sadness. Sickness or fatigue, difficulties in problem-solving, threats of loss of love or any occasion of loneliness become doubly difficult to tolerate when shame is added to the sadness. Under such conditions the individual is constantly prompted to apologise for his own existence, heaping contempt upon himself and others whenever anything is in any way distressing. He may further try to avoid such experiences by denying that there is any reason either for himself or others to feel distress. Such an individual will find it doubly difficult to tolerate physical pain or frustration in problem-solving or loneliness.

EMOTIONAL UNAWARENESS: DEFENCE OR DEFICIT?

Mr Baker's symptoms disappeared after the second consultation and he gave the credit for his improvement to drinking a glass of sparkling water. Later, reflecting on our interaction, I realised that I felt not only impatient with his lack of insight, but also disappointed because I experienced his remark as devaluing my therapeutic work. Fortunately, I knew that the doctor who has adopted a psychodynamic approach to a patient who is emotionally unaware might experience the patient's lack of emotional understanding as a personal rejection. It is recognised that offering psychotherapeutic help to patients who are not psychologically minded can activate negative feelings in the doctor who, in his turn, might adopt an attitude of rejection or adhere defensively to a purely organic approach (Taylor 1976). Therapists have retaliated by calling such people heart-sink patients (O'Dowd 1988), normopaths (McDougall 1980a), antianalysands (McDougall 1980b), normotics (Bollas 1987), immature personalities (Ruesch 1948) and emotional illiterates (Freedman and Sweet 1954). Their emotional unawareness has thwarted conventional psychotherapeutic approaches and has become the focus of intensive research.

When I first met Mr Baker, his unawareness of grief made me think that he possessed the alexithymic personality characteristics. I therefore administered the TAS-20 questionnaire and was very surprised to realise not only that his TAS-20 score was well within the normal range but also that it had not changed at all since the first time he had taken it two years previously when he had developed shingles. I wondered initially whether he did not answer the questionnaire honestly in order to present me with a better image of himself; whether his difficulty with emotion concerned only the affect of distress and therefore was not picked up by the questionnaire; or whether it was only the presence of his doctor, an authority figure to whom he could not admit his sadness.

In retrospect, however, I think that the result accurately reflected his ability to weep and therefore his potential to get in touch with his feelings and benefit from a psychodynamic approach. In this case I consider that his emotional unawareness was the result of a repressive defensive style rather than alexithymia, a stable personality trait that consists of a cluster of deficits in the capacity to process emotions cognitively and symbolically. Obviously this is a fascinating area for research in general practice. It may help in choosing the right therapeutic approach for emotionally unaware patients.

THE IMPORTANCE OF EMOTIONAL AWARENESS FOR DEVELOPING THE CAPACITY TO MOURN

Freud has identified mourning as a psychic process, a normal function of bereaved individuals, that helps them to master the feelings of grief and come to terms with their loss (Freud 1917). Helene Deutsch, in her classic paper 'Absence of grief', maintained that mourning strives for realisation, and that the unresolved process of mourning must in some way be expressed in full. The expediency of the flight from the suffering of grief by omitting the emotional response is but a temporary gain because Deutsch believed that the necessity to mourn persists in the psyche (Deutsch 1937).

However, Krystal (1988) has emphasised that there are certain prerequisites for the capacity to mourn. First of all, there is a limit to the kind and number of losses an individual can deal with successfully, for example how much loss the survivors of the Holocaust could absorb through grieving. Also, good affect tolerance is needed in order to carry out the process of mourning without it snowballing into a maladaptive state of depression. The affects that are tolerated best are of adult type, are not overwhelming, with minimal physiological components, are mostly idea-like and can be used as information to the self. Adult affects are the result of extensive cognitive processing and symbolic elaboration of emotional arousal. It follows that a requirement for successful mourning is an awareness of and a capacity to tolerate grief.

HELPING THE PATIENT TO DEVELOP EMOTIONAL AWARENESS

The act of labelling emotions can have a soothing effect on the nervous system, helping the patient to recover more quickly from emotionally upsetting incidents (Pennebaker 1985, Pennebaker and Susman 1988). Thus the doctor can be of great help to the patient by adopting an emotion coaching attitude (see also Chapter 5) and assisting him in his handling of both the physical and emotional aspects of affects. Patients need to become acquainted with their emotions as signals, often unpleasant but manageable and essentially self-limited. In this respect, the doctor belatedly supplies a function that the patient's parents failed to perform. Like a teacher, the therapist should help the patient learn to recognise, label, interpret and organise his own feelings.

Although there is an analogy between the parental role and that of the general practitioner as providers of total care for their children and their patients respectively, the doctor needs to have acquired a special skill if he is to engage in emotion coaching with his patients. He must have undergone some emotion coaching himself, and he must have achieved some degree of emotional intelligence. The foundation of emotion coaching is the capacity for empathy. It is the ability to put ourselves in other people's shoes and imagine how we would feel in their place. It is the ability to recognise and understand other people's feelings. The doctor can appreciate the emotional experience of others only in the context of an ongoing differentiated awareness of his own, and only if he is capable of adequate reflective self-awareness and sensitive self-observation. Unless he is able to recognise his own emotional states, to name them accurately and to use them as information to himself, he may not be in a position to listen empathically to his patient's feelings. The empathic listener uses his heart to feel what his patient is feeling, uses his eyes to watch for physical evidence of his patient's emotions, and his imagination to see the situation from his patient's perspective. He uses the latter's words to reflect back in a soothing uncritical way what he is hearing and helps his patient to label his own emotions.

I was able to engage in emotion coaching with Mr Baker, which I believe contributed to an understanding and a resolution of his symptoms, only because of all the information I had gathered in six twenty-minute consultations over a period of two years. This in turn was possible because of my interest in problems of emotional communication and expression and readiness to become emotionally engaged by creating the space to unfold a relatively relaxed discussion.

CONCLUSION

In our busy surgeries we are faced every day with patients who complain of symptoms which we cannot easily diagnose during our brief encounter with them. Within five minutes or less, all we can do is find out what they are afraid may be wrong with them and (if to do so is appropriate) reassure them that their symptoms and our clinical findings do not support their fear. In other words, we can tell them only what they do *not* suffer from, but we cannot make a positive diagnosis.

Some patients seem to be satisfied with the reassurance that we can find nothing seriously wrong with their bodies, but a few will insist on finding out the exact cause of their suffering. This is a crucial moment in the consultation, the handling of which depends on a variety of factors and which can determine the subsequent relationship of the patient with the doctor. There is a danger that if the doctor is overwhelmed and harassed by the many patients pressing to be seen immediately who are not particularly psychologically minded, his motivation may change from sympathetic understanding of the patient to personal survival. Under these circumstances, he may respond dismissively by fobbing the patient off with a plausible diagnosis, or a prescription, or adhering rigidly to a biomedical model which can only lead to more and more tests in search of an elusive disease. This activity might or might not confirm the patient's fears that he is suffering from a fatal condition that is difficult to diagnose (Halton 1995). Alternately, the doctor can play for time, order some tests and invite the patient to return at a quieter time for a longer appointment. It may be possible then to use this time as an opportunity for emotion coaching. Such an approach makes it possible to pay attention to the patient's cues of both his conscious and unconscious agenda, encouraging him to identify his concerns, fears and expectations, and express them in words that accurately identify his emotional state. When these conditions prevail, it may be possible to help the patient recognise that certain physical sensations are the direct consequence of experiencing his emotions.

13 'IF THINE EYE OFFEND THEE, PLUCK IT OUT'*

EYES AND FEELINGS

Of all the afflictions of the body, those of the eye arouse the greatest fear in patients and their general practitioners. Because the fear of blindness can be stronger than the fear of death (Fitzgerald 1970), doctors tend to refer patients with eye problems to the ophthalmologist sooner rather than later. This fear may be partly responsible for a lack of awareness that some eye problems can be influenced by emotions. Medical students and some doctors are surprised when I mention that weeping is one of the most frequent psychosomatic symptoms. And yet the eyes are central to the expression and experience of emotions. Not only are they part of the face where all human emotions are displayed and communicated and therefore they are involved in crying, but also primitive affect precursors may be experienced as iconic visual images. It seems that the visual representation of certain emotional states has a greater impact on the body than a verbal account of them. Vrana and his colleagues have provided experimental support for this hypothesis by demonstrating that visual imagination of a feared situation leads to physiological activation, whereas verbal articulation of the same material leads to little or no arousal (Vrana et al. 1986). This finding is in keeping with the developmental view of affects according to which unregulated and primitive emotions before they are cognitively processed and mastered are experienced as physical sensations and action tendencies. It also points the way to the treatment of these patients which should be helping them to recognise their emotions and talk about them in a way that leads to their cognitive processing and mastery.

The importance of considering emotional difficulties in disorders of the eye was first brought to my attention in 1992 by Alexis Brook, a psychoanalytic psychotherapist, during a talk about his research at the annual Balint dinner in 1992. Dr Brook who has an interest in psychosomatic medicine and is experienced in psychological problems in general practice (Brook et al. 1966, Brook and Temperley 1976) was already involved in research on psychosomatic eye disorders at the opthalmic department of Queen Alexandra Hospital in Portsmouth (Brook 1995).This is the hospital where William

---

* Matthew 5: 29.

Inman, a pioneer ophthalmic surgeon who had also trained as a psychoanalyst had worked at the beginning of the twentieth century. He had written many original papers on the relationship between emotional conflicts and eye conditions, the best known of which was 'Styes, barley and wedding rings' (Inman 1946, 1964).

I was fascinated by Brook's project, and a few days after I had expressed my enthusiasm about his work he contacted me in order to explore the possibility of extending his research to general practice. This was a once-in-a-lifetime opportunity. My partners and I invited him to come to the Well Street surgery once a fortnight to see patients with eye disorders that we would be referring to him. This was the beginning of a very fruitful and interesting collaboration which continues to the time of writing (March 2000).

We decided to begin by focusing on blepharitis because, of all eye conditions, blepharitis is the least likely to threaten vision and therefore the most likely to be managed entirely in the general practice setting. It is an inflammatory or infective condition of the eyelids that does not always respond to conventional medical treatment and tends to become chronic or to recur. In twenty consecutive sufferers we found an association between chronic recurring blepharitis and prolonged grieving. But perhaps the most striking finding was that more than half the patients had suffered severe losses in infancy or childhood. It is possible that such early loss might have been difficult to accept and might have led to difficulties in adapting to further losses later in life and a tendency to chronic grieving (Brook and Zalidis 1999).

In 1995 Alexis Brook and I were invited by Andrew Elder, a general practitioner who at the time was also a consultant in General Practice at the Tavistock Clinic, to plan a multidisciplinary research seminar to study more widely how emotional problems influence the eye.

The members of this first historic eye research seminar, which ran for twenty sessions, were recruited from a variety of disciplines. Apart from the three leaders, we had one other general practitioner, two eye surgeons, a paediatric ophthalmologist, two ophthalmic social workers, two orthoptists and two optometrists. The results of this work were presented in 'The mind's eye', a symposium held at Moorfields Eye Hospital in October 1997 (Brook et al. 1998).

My contribution was an examination of the emotional context within which two patients developed severe eye pain. It was this interest in psychosomatic eye disorders that helped to contain my own and my patients' fear of blindness long enough to take a detailed history, and find out the circumstances preceding the pain, that made sense of the symptom and provided the treatment at the same time (Zalidis 1998b).

EYE PAIN AS A WARNING OF IMPENDING DANGER

Most cases of eye pain remain medically unexplained and may be referred to as functional syndromes or somatoform disorders. However, this does not mean that they are 'all in the mind'. So-called functional symptoms occur in the context of emotional arousal and the contemporary way of under-standing emotions recognises that they are simultaneously biological and psychological phenomena. In this theoretical framework most functional somatic symptoms can be explained by the physiological mechanisms that mediate emotional arousal.

In the disregulation model of psychosomatic medicine (see Chapter 3) pain may be understood as a direct manifestation of unregulated emotion and thus a symptom of somatisation. Our understanding of pain has changed recently and pain theorists view pain as an abnormal affective state and not as a primary perceptual experience. It has been suggested that chronic pain can be viewed as a third pathologic emotion interfacing closely with anxiety and depression and that it has its own neurochemical correlates in the integrative centres of the brain (Swanson 1984). Graeme Taylor and his colleagues, extending this hypothesis, argued that acute pain can be viewed as a signal affect serving a protective function comparable to those of signal anxiety and signal depression. It warns the self about impending dangers and about the possible need to mobilise defences to deal with them. Such dangers may include the emergence of a much more unpleasant emotion, loss of love, loss of self-esteem, the threat of mutilation, and so on (Taylor 1987). The following case histories will provide examples of such threats.

Christopher

Christopher, a twenty-five-year old, presented to the surgery complaining that for the last three days he was experiencing sharp shooting pains in his left eye. This was the second episode of eye pain in a year. Because he had damaged his right eye six years previously he was worried that if anything happened to his good eye he would effectively become blind. He had already complained to his optician who had suggested that the pain was due to the muscles of the left eye straining to compensate for the damaged right eye. He was not satisfied with this explanation, however, because he had not had pains from the start of the injury to the right eye six years ago.

General practitioners often have the advantage of knowing the medical history of the other members of a patient's family. A year previously, Christo-pher's mother had had coronary artery bypass surgery and she became seriously ill from complications. During the operation she developed acute ischaemia of the right leg due to femoral artery dissection, which caused the muscles to swell. In order to relieve the pressure the surgeons made a cut in the muscle envelope, which later had to be extended. The wound became infected. Because I heard Christopher say that the first episode of eye pain had occurred a year ago, around the time of his mother's operation, I mentioned her illness. To my surprise he remembered that he had experienced the eye pain for the first time after a visit to the hospital where his mother had shown him her damaged leg.

When I asked him how he had felt when he saw it, he looked at me, wrinkled his nose, lifted his upper lip, protruded his lower lip and tongue and said that he felt disgusted. He immediately turned his eyes away in revulsion. He could not look. The leg was opened up as if somebody had hacked it with a machete. The eye pain started as soon as he walked away.

After that visit he could not bear to look at his mother's leg, which is still marked by the extensive scars of the operation, because the scars remind him of his disgust at the hospital. However, since his mother returned home she has been asking him to put emollient cream on the hard skin of her feet and he begs her every time not to remove her support stockings so that he will not have to look at the scars.

I asked if anything had happened three days ago to bring back the visual memories of his mother's leg. He remembered that the pain started after a conversation with his mother during which she told him that the surgeons had advised her to have a below-knee amputation of the injured leg. The muscles had become fibrosed and the nerves damaged, and this made walking very difficult for her. He immediately felt alarmed and begged her not to let them amputate her leg. The pain followed soon after.

Jonathan

One day towards the end of March, Jonathan was the last patient on my list and so I did not have to force the pace of his consultation. He was dressed in a smart suit, utilising his waiting time by doing some paperwork he had with him in his briefcase. He looked serious and taciturn. He complained of aching behind the right eye which produced a nauseous feeling. The pain started gradually, reached a peak and disappeared within three or four hours. At the peak of the pain his vision became a bit blurred. The pain usually started between noon and 4 o'clock in the afternoon, including weekends. He told me rather briskly that he was used to working under a lot of pressure, wanting obviously to forestall any facile suggestions that his pain was due to stress at work. He assured me that his pain was very strong and that he was not one to make a fuss. It was his wife who insisted that he came to see the doctor. After taking the history of the complaint I went on to take a family history. When I asked whether his mother was healthy, he told me that she was healthy when she died!

I was surprised by this revelation and pressed him for more information. He told me that she had died in a road traffic accident at the beginning of April twenty-four years ago at the age of forty-four. I asked him how old he was, and he told me that he would be forty-four in a few days, at the beginning of April. I was astonished.

After a physical examination of the eye and his face, I could not find any abnormality and so I told him that the most striking finding was the triple anniversary. In a week's time, on the anniversary of his mother's death, almost on his birthday, he would become the age at which his mother had died.

It was his turn to be surprised. He was not aware that he was reaching the age at which his mother had died, but he was quick to deny that he was worrying about anything like that. He had got over her death and it was all in the past. He looked at me rather sternly and said that he was not an emotional person and that he had too many responsibilities to be concerned with emotional matters.

I acknowledged that he was not an emotional person, and also that it was my duty to point out to him that in my experience people do develop symptoms on the anniversary of the death of an important person in their lives. I asked him how he felt when his mother died, and he said that he was inconsolable for three weeks (he was twenty years old when his mother died).

I suggested that the pain had something to do with stress caused by his mother's death, the memory of which had been reactivated by the triple anniversary. If his symptoms did not improve in the next few days he should come back for further investigation. He told me that he was satisfied with my thorough examination and that he expected the pain to clear if it was indeed related to the anniversaries.

I did not hear from him again until a couple of years later when I received a request to write an insurance report about him. It was obvious from the notes that he had not seen another doctor in the meantime. It is a fair assumption that his symptoms had cleared and he remained healthy.

DISGUST AS A SIGNAL OF FEELINGS OF REJECTION

Because it has been shown that verbal communication of affective distress reduces autonomic arousal and appears to protect against somatic symptom formation, I encourage my patients to talk about the way they feel. I find that patients have varying degrees of difficulty in identifying and naming their emotional states, and so I was rather surprised when Christopher identified his disgust so unequivocally. What is disgust, and how could it be related to eye pain?

For Darwin the term 'disgust' in its simplest sense meant something offensive to the taste (Darwin 1872). From an evolutionary point of view, disgust has the adaptive function of protecting us from harmful foods by limiting our hunger and pulling us away from whatever triggered it. In other words, disgust started life as a biological defence. Silvan Tomkins, the founder of affect theory (see Chapter 3), called disgust initially an affect auxiliary because it is programmed to limit the drive of hunger, at least temporarily, and to ensure that either the offending substance is expelled with vigour or that we distance ourselves from it (Tomkins 1963). However, during development, disgust has acquired the function of a signal, to the self and to others, of feelings of rejection. The awareness of disgust is no longer limited to offensive tastes but is elicited by a wide spectrum of entities that need not be tasted or ingested. In Western culture, taste has become a metaphor for an aesthetic and social sense of discernment, and whatever offends our aesthetic or moral sense can activate our disgust.

For this reason Tomkins, in his later work, included disgust in his list of the six negative innate emotions. Disgust is a strong word that can evoke a sense of alarm and shock and it is much more than distaste. Disgust is an emotion. Disgust is what revolts and repels us. Disgust involves intrusive and persistent thoughts about the repugnance at the object that triggered it. Disgust is accompanied by ideas and images of danger. The danger of pollution and contamination. The danger of defilement. We believe that anything that comes into contact with the disgusting becomes tainted and acquires the capacity to disgust. Even writing about disgust is to risk contamination, and I hope readers will forgive me for exposing them to the risk of contamination, too!

Like all innate affects, disgust is characterised by a unique facial expression which involves wrinkling the nose, raising the upper lip, protruding the lower lip and the tongue. The 'Yuck!' response. It may also be accompanied by its physiological markers of nausea and vomiting and characteristic spitting, cringing and recoil.

IS EYE PAIN RELATED TO VISUALLY EVOKED DISGUST?

The fact that disgust is very much related to the gut and has been called the most visceral of all emotions has distracted us from realising that other senses are involved in evoking disgust.

The social historian William Miller, in a brilliant book on disgust, has pointed out that before the word entered the English vocabulary in the first quarter of the seventeenth century, taste figured distinctly less prominently than foul odours and loathsome sights (Miller 1997). Tomkins has coined the word 'dissmell' to indicate a response analogous to disgust which is elicited by offensive smells (Tomkins 1963), but we have no equivalent word to indicate response to disgusting sights, loathsome visual images and repulsive visual memories.

Vision is the sense through which much of horror is accessed. Horror is a complex affective state, a combination of disgust and fear. Although disgust has a range of intensity from relatively mild to strong, horror is always an intense experience. Mild horror is no longer horror. There are few things that are more unnerving and evocative of disgust than mutilations and the violation of the body envelope. Consider the horror we experience at the sight of victims of landmines with amputated legs, visual images of beheading, or severely mutilated victims of road traffic accidents. It is sight that processes ugliness, deformity, mutilation and most of what we perceive as violence, such as carnage, indignities and violations. The visual has its own sense of aesthetic and consequent moral standards which if breached can evoke disgust, pity and fear. Amputation is horrifying no matter what part is detached. According to Miller the danger comes from identification with the victim.

Paradoxically the disgusting also has allure. It attracts as well as repels exerting a fascination that manifests itself in the difficulty of averting our eyes at a gory accident. The paparazzi trying to photograph the dying Diana,

Princess of Wales, in her wrecked car were responding to this allure. Plato gives an example of this fascination in *The Republic*.

It is a story about a young Athenian, Leontion the son of Aglaion, who was on his way to Athens from Piraeus, under the outer side of the north wall, when he noticed some corpses lying on the ground with the executioner standing by them. He wanted to go and look at them, and yet at the same time held himself back in disgust. For a time he struggled with himself and covered his eyes, but at last his desire got the better of him and he ran up to the corpses, opening his eyes wide and saying to them: There you are curse you- a lovely sight! Have a real good look!

Plato does not mention whether the exposure to the disgusting sight was followed by an attack of eye pain, but perhaps Leontion's positive emotion of interest protected him by modulating his negative emotions of disgust and anger.

When we are confronted by a loathsome sight we can avoid it by averting our gaze or closing our eyes. However, when we are haunted by a disgusting visual memory or visual images there is no escape.

Christopher experienced disgust when he first saw the loathsome sight of his mother's wounds, and he developed eye pain soon afterwards. Since then he protected himself from re-experiencing disgust by insisting that his mother kept her support stockings on to hide the scars. He developed the second episode of eye pain after his mother told him that she was considering having her leg amputated. This conversation threatened to reactivate his disgust at the loathsome visual memory of her damaged leg, and his fear that some part of his own body might be amputated too.

The importance of the emotion of disgust for the development of Jonathan's eye pain is less obvious. I can only speculate that as his unconscious identification with his mother was reaching its peak at the approach of the triple anniversary, the possible reactivation of horrific images of her injured body could have evoked disgust that motivated the rejection of these images and the accompanying grief.

Another possible trigger for the arousal of disgust is related to Miller's observation that the display of any emotion considered to be a breach of decorum can activate disgust. It is possible that Jonathan's memory of his inconsolability after his mother's death could have seemed to him excessive and childish and therefore unseemly, to the point of activating self-disgust or even shame. His hostile reaction to my emotion coaching attitude and his assertion that he had too many responsibilities to be concerned with emotional matters lends some support to this hypothesis.

CONCLUSION

Although the role of disgust in several psychiatric conditions has recently been recognised (Philips et al. 1998), more research is needed in order to ascertain whether eye pain is the somatic expression of visually activated disgust. In both cases, however, it is possible to understand eye pain as a signal, warning that horrific images accompanying primitive and over-whelming emotions are about to be activated and that the patient has to guard against them, to blind himself as it were, to disgusting images, loathsome sights and negative emotions. This way of understanding eye pain brings us full circle to Matthew's advice: 'If thine eye offend thee, pluck it out', which demonstrates an intuitive understanding of the problems discussed in this chapter, even though the emotional state alluded to by the Apostle is forbidden lust rather than horror and grief.

14   CONTINUITY OF CARE

The four essentials of primary care have been defined as accessibility, comprehensiveness, coordination and continuity of care (McWhinney 1998a). Despite increasing pressures on general practice to screen for risk factors and early disease in asymptomatic individuals, for most general practitioners the key relationship continues to be with individual patients who consult about problems they have identified for themselves. General practice still represents a strong tradition of personal care, comprehensive in its response to the needs of the people and reasonably accessible in their neighbourhoods and homes.

It is said that in hospital medicine, persons come and go and diseases stay, whereas in general practice, diseases come and go and persons stay. Traditionally, the commitment of the general practitioner is to the person and not to the patient with a certain disease. General practice defines itself in terms of relationships and not in terms of diseases or technologies. The commitment is ongoing and ended only by retirement, death or a decision to end the relationship by either party. The key role of the general practitioner is to respond to the initial presentation of illness, to respond to suffering and make a clinical assessment. Ian McWhinney, Professor of Family Medicine at the University of Ontario, has emphasised that compassion is not conditional on evidence of its effectiveness and that responding to suffering is a moral obligation (McWhinney 1998b). He thinks that a general practitioner's relationship with his patient is better described as a covenant rather than a contract which sets out the limits of what can be expected of the parties. A contract says: 'I am committed to doing so much, but not more.' A covenant is an undertaking to do whatever is needed.

However, sticking with a person though thick and thin is hard work and may test the ability of the doctor to tolerate painful emotions to the limit.

ROSE

Skin Language

I first met Rose and her family in August 1987. They asked for my help with Rose's mother, Mrs K, whose behaviour was causing problems. Mrs K used to live alone until her progressing dementia made her so confused that she could not find her way back home, or count the correct change. Her youngest daughter, Rose, and Rose's husband, Mark, decided to take her into their home and look after her. Rose, who was a security guard in an old people's home at the time, was the breadwinner. Mark stayed at home and cared for their two-year-old daughter, Rachel, and Mrs K. They decided on this arrangement because Rose's job was the better paid.

Looking after Mrs K, however, proved a very difficult task. She was a heavy smoker and she burnt holes in the carpets and the curtains. She was incontinent of urine and very often she would refuse to wear her incontinence pads. She would urinate on the carpet in her bedroom and would leave her dirty underwear on the kitchen draining board. She would have fights with Mark when he insisted that she had a bath, abuse him verbally and accuse him of being physically violent. Very often she would ask him what was he doing in her own house. Her behaviour was deteriorating and on a few occasions she went out and got lost and the police had to find her and bring her back. Mark found her behaviour infuriating and asked me to see her in the hope that she suffered from a curable illness. All the tests were normal, however, and the psycho-geriatrician who examined her confirmed that she was suffering from Alzheimer's dementia. In view of her offensive behaviour he arranged regular day hospital attendance and put her on the waiting list for admission to a psycho-geriatric ward.

Rose came to see me a month after my initial involvement with her mother. She was then forty-four years old, very thin, with short black hair. She had a deep masculine voice which contrasted with Mark's youthful voice, which sounded almost feminine. She complained of feeling awful. She had constant headaches, was sleeping badly, her appetite was poor and she was losing weight. Rose found that when her mother had a temper tantrum at home, she also reacted to her mother's past violence. Mrs K had treated her children in a harsh way which amounted almost to physical abuse. Rose had always lived in fear of her mother who regularly beat and threatened her with abandonment. Her eldest sister went deaf in one ear when her mother banged her head against a wall in a fit of rage.

She told me that one of her greatest fears now was that Mark might crack up under the strain of her mother's behaviour. She had reason to fear this because four months after their wedding, Mark had stolen all her money and jewellery and disappeared for several days. He had binged on intravenous heroin, during which he contracted hepatitis B and then infected her. Fortunately, they both recovered and Mark had never repeated his behaviour, but Rose was afraid that the present stress at home might precipitate a recurrence. Meanwhile, Mark was showing his distress by withdrawing his help and taking to his bed. Rose was so obviously distressed that I asked her to come and see me weekly for support.

The situation at home deteriorated, and so did Rose's symptoms. She was aching all over and was crying constantly. She developed generalised itching which later became localised to the pubic area. On examination the skin was red and raw, with scratch marks oozing blood. As I could see no parasites, I prescribed calamine lotion – a cooling, soothing skin preparation – which had no effect whatsoever.

Mrs K's condition deteriorated quickly and in January 1988 she became unable to get out of bed. I admitted her to hospital where she died one month later.

One week after her mother's death, Rose came to the surgery saying that she needed to talk about her mother. Also, the rash in her pubic area had spread to involve the whole hypogastrium. The itching was so intense that she wanted to tear herself to pieces. She said that she was terrified of the dark. She thought that this might have something to do with her mother telling her that when she died she would come and haunt her. She felt guilty about her mother's death because she let the doctors give her pethidine, a strong opioid painkiller which can make you drowsy, to relieve her agony during the last hours of her life. This probably made her die sooner than expected and Rose had the feeling that she had killed her. One day at the hospital she was struggling to change her mother's nightie when Mrs K started shouting: 'Don't hit me, don't hit me.' Rose felt she could not cope any longer. 'You have been doing all the hitting', she shouted, and she ran away. Mark had to take over.

Because the rash was not getting any better I assumed that it was caused by a candida infection to which she was allergic and I prescribed Nystatin, an anti-candida cream, and antihistamines. I also made a mental note of the link between the desire to tear herself to pieces and her account of the hitting mother.

One week later Rose came again. Her itching and the rash were as intense as ever. She talked and cried throughout the consultation. She said that she knew when she was little that her mother could not cope with life for whatever reason, and that Rose made her mother's life that bit more difficult. When her mother was angry she would threaten to leave her and Rose would beg her not to. The more she begged the more threatening her mother became. Then she would get violent headaches and beat her. Rose used to pray that she got the headaches instead so that her mother would be in a better mood. Her mother would not let her cry. If she cried, she would beat her and so she had to pretend she was not crying. When her mother was in hospital Rose wanted to tell her that she always cared for her, but she could not say anything until her mother was unconscious and could not hear her; otherwise she was afraid that her mother might say something terrible. Rose had never been able to show her mother any tender feelings without her mother shouting abuse at her. Just before she died, she opened her eyes and looked at Rose in a terrifying way as if she was blaming her for everything. Rose cried because she never got what she wanted from her mother: love, companionship and care.

A week later Rose's itching was no better, despite my various remedies. Her fear that her mother would come and haunt her was so strong that she had to leave all the lights on. When she brushed her teeth in the bathroom she had to face the door in case her mother appeared behind her back. Her fear infected me and I became worried that her excoriated skin was invaded by secondaries from an undiagnosed carcinoma. I began to wonder whether I should refer her for a specialist opinion. However, I contained my anxiety and told her very tentatively that I thought her itching had something to do with her relationship to her mother. 'Yes', she replied. 'Sackcloth and ashes.'

A week after this cryptic comment, Rose came to the surgery looking very well. She was elegantly dressed, had a confident, happy look about her and was almost beautiful. She reported that during the past week she had had two dreams, following which she felt a lot better. Her itchy rash had gone.

In the first dream she was running through wide roads. A man called her to follow him. She had to make her way through brambles. Suddenly she came to the end of the brambles where there was a precipice and she fell. The fall caused a pressure in her chest and she woke up very frightened.

In the second dream she felt there was something final about her mother's death. Rose was looking for her daughter and could not find her. She was shouting and screaming, calling for her. Mark very calmly said that she was all right, she was asleep. She woke up in terror and she went to check if Rachel was all right.

I interpreted to her that the brambles that tore her skin represented her relationship to her cruel mother. When her mother died and the brambles came to an end there was nothing to support her and she fell. It was either brambles or nothing. All her life she was terrified that her mother might leave her, and finally she had.

The second dream expressed her terror that along with the brambles – the bad mother – she might lose the good mother, represented by her relationship to her daughter, and be left utterly alone. This would be intolerable and she had to reassure herself in real life that her daughter was still there. These two dreams expressed Rose's problems in a nutshell: her clinging for comfort to a mother who inflicted pain, so that comfort and pain became inseparable.

Mark Gets Under Her Skin

After the resolution of her rash, Rose continued to attend the surgery two or three times a month for various minor complaints of her own or for Rachel. She also changed jobs and became a pest control officer. This involved handling insecticides and poisons. In January 1989, one year after the first appearance of her itchy rash, it reappeared. She complained that her pubic area was so itchy that she was tearing herself to shreds. She scratched so hard that she made herself bleed. The appearance of the rash was identical to that of the previous year. I reminded her that last time she had had a similar problem she was very upset about her mother's illness and I wondered if there was anything upsetting her this time. She was upset about Mark. He was in one of his foul moods. He was withdrawn, angry and swore at her. She was frightened of his verbal abuse. Also, he was not reliable with Rachel and she had to take dependency leave to look after her for the time being. She was worried that if Mark did not get out of this frame of mind she would have to find a childminder, and she hated this possibility. She was not sure whether Mark was taking drugs and she was afraid that if she told him that everything was over between them, then he might take Rachel and disappear.

Then she said that Mark had got under her skin recently. I wondered out loud whether in a sense she was attacking him where she thought she could find him; that is, under her skin. This comment did not make much of an impression. I examined her hypogastrium and prescribed some calamine lotion and an antihistamine. A fortnight later she returned and said: 'The itching is driving me doolally.' She wanted literally to tear herself to pieces. She finally found a childminder who would look after Rachel while Rose was at work. She did not trust Mark when he went into his moods. She found that Rachel was unsupervised, and watched a lot of television. One day she came home earlier than usual and found the Christmas tree stripped bare of the chocolates she had put on it. The electric lights were next to them and Mark did not notice that Rachel could have been electrocuted. She told him how disappointed she was that he did not look after her properly and ended up crying, and she hated it.

I asked whether she was angry with him for not keeping his side of the agreement. She answered indirectly by saying that she pitied him and felt sorry for him. She said that it was Mark who was full of hatred; that he was like a bag of pus. He felt sorry for himself and behaved well for a while, but now and then the bag exploded and all the pus came out on to her face. I asked whether this hatred made her angry. She evaded my question by saying she did not like it when he showered her with verbal abuse. I interpreted to her that her itching was her way of expressing anger. But she said that was silly because in that way she only hurt herself. I explained to her that she turned her anger against herself. Her mother had seen to that. It was never safe to show her anger when she was little because she was punished severely. Now her mother lived inside her. To my amazement she started crying and said that she had been missing her mother a lot lately. When she took her into her home to look after her she had hoped that she could change her.

As the itching was so severe and had not responded to my previous remedies I prescribed hydrocortisone, a mild steroidal anti-inflammatory cream, and asked her to come again the following week. When she arrived she was smiling and looked relaxed. She complained of a tummy upset and a lump behind the ear. Not a word about the itching. In the end I could wait no longer and I asked her about it. She astonished me by saying that her aunt told her to put surgical spirit on it. It hurt a lot at first but then it got better.

'You see', said Rose defiantly; 'all the creams and oily stuff that you gave me warm the skin and make the itching worse.'

Rose had not given me any credit for the improvement of her itchy rash. It was only two years later when I was writing Rose's story that I realised that on both occasions her rash improved after I had interpreted its possible meaning to her. It is difficult to know in retrospect what was the therapeutic factor. Was it my acknowledgement of the anger that she externalised on Mark, or giving her the opportunity to talk freely about her distress? We know that when we do not make it possible for patients to tell us about the abuse they have suffered, we fulfil their transference expectations of our being uncaring mothers.

Rose's Experience of Anger is Blocked by Fear

After the resolution of the second episode of her rash, Rose continued to attend frequently: sometimes once a month; sometimes three times a month. Her dissatisfaction with Mark's behaviour increased.

In April 1989 she had an accident at work. A puff of Drione powder, one of the insecticides she was using, touched her face. She came to see me for advice. I contacted the poison centre at Guy's Hospital. The specialist did not think it was serious. After this incident, Rose's complaints increased in frequency and intensity. She developed back pain for which I referred her to the physiotherapy department. She developed pain in her elbow due to inflammation of the area where the tendon enters the bone, which I injected with a steroidal anti-inflammatory drug. She developed irregular menstrual periods for which I referred her to a gynaecologist who put her on the waiting list for a dilatation and curettage.

In February 1990 she complained of feeling chronically tired. She felt exhausted and found her job physically demanding. She enjoyed the mental part concerning the knowledge of the lifecycle of the various pests, but not the physical part which entailed killing them. She was aching all over and felt sick. Her mouth filled with saliva, she vomited and then felt absolutely drained. At the end of the consultation she added: 'My aunt told me to make sure I have my blood pressure and my blood checked.'

I remembered the beneficial effect her aunt had had on her from the second episode of her itchy rash and wanted to ally myself with her. I told Rose that I had the greatest respect for her aunt, and then examined her and ordered several tests in order to help with the differential diagnosis. Every test was normal, but her complaints became relentless and dramatic. She hurt all over and felt as if her bones were falling to pieces. She felt so exhausted that one morning she was halfway to work and had to turn her car around to go back home. She felt she had run out of whatever it was that had sustained her since Mark ran away with her jewellery and had a drug binge six years ago. She asked me to refer her for homoeopathic treatment. I had no objection, but while she was waiting for an outpatient appointment I thought that she needed some urgent help. I told her that I did not think she was suffering from a physical disease but that she was very unhappy. I asked her whether she would like to come and see me each week for twenty minutes until my summer holiday in three weeks time, and she accepted.

In our first session, she told me that she was physically in agony but could not afford to be ill. She had lost her self-respect. She had lost respect for Mark. She felt nothing for him. Nothing to build on. She felt sorry for him. She felt grateful to him for giving her Rachel, who is hers. I asked her whether she was angry with Mark. She told me that she cannot experience anger. She cannot even feel angry with her mother. She told me again how, when she was little, she used to pray that she got the headaches instead of her mother, because her mother used to give her a hiding with a belt every time she got a headache. These memories were painful and Rose started crying. She even used to buy powders to cure her mother's headaches, but her mother would still beat her. When her mother was ill at home, she asked why had she beaten her all the time. The mother replied that somebody had to do it. Rose said that she had put all these painful memories in little boxes but she cannot keep them locked away for too long.

A week later Rose was feeling no better. The day before she came to see me, Mark had been aggressive and had ended up swearing at her. Rose was appalled at how subservient she became during the row. She blamed herself subsequently for getting in Mark's way. I felt that this was the right moment for an interpretation. 'So from what you are saying it seems that when Mark is aggressive to you, he becomes your angry mother and you become the frightened little girl. You lose your adulthood and therefore your self respect.' This interpretation brought up a flood of memories about her relationship to her mother. From as far back as Rose could remember, her mother had beaten her. She could not reason with her mother, just as she cannot reason with Mark when he is in one of his moods. She was molested at the age of seven by a mentally defective neighbour who asked her to touch him. When her mother found out about this from her brother she beat her, because she said that it was her fault. When her periods were late at the age of thirteen, her mother took her to a specialist and swore that she was pregnant.

'How frightening it must have been for you', I said.

'Yes', she replied, ' I was brought up in fear. If Mark ever hits Rachel, he will find himself out of the front door before his feet touch the ground.'

The following week Rose was still very tired, but she began making some startling discoveries. She felt guilty for taking so many weeks off work. She was afraid that her boss would not believe that she was ill. She asked her aunt's advice, who told her that it did not really matter whether her boss believed her or not. When she told her boss over the telephone that she did not feel fit to come back to work yet, she was surprised about how easily she accepted it. She realised that she expected to be told off all the time. Never before had she associated her feelings with her mother's behaviour. Her mother never believed her. When she was playing with her sister and brother and someone cried, it was always her fault and she got a beating. When her periods started she was totally unprepared for the experience. She soiled her underwear with blood and was terrified that her mother would beat her for this. When she was taken to a surgeon to have a cyst removed from her face, the mother did not warn her of the impending operation. When she recovered from the anaesthetic she had excruciating pain in her throat. The surgeon told her mother that as her breathing was noisy, he had also removed her tonsils and adenoids. As a consequence the bill was higher than expected, and her mother was annoyed with Rose for not breathing quietly under the anaesthetic. 'Even when I was asleep I was in the wrong', said Rose wryly. Suddenly the thought that her expectations of people's reactions to her had been conditioned by her mother's behaviour and did not correspond to present-day situations was a revelation and a liberation. This was our last session before my holiday, and I was going to be surprised when I came back.

Rose Develops the Capacity to Soothe Her Body

She came to see me as soon as I returned from holiday. She told me that she had not been able to wait for the homoeopathic appointment to come through and so during my absence she had gone privately to a nature clinic. There she was seen first by a homoeopathic doctor. As soon as he heard that she was working with insecticides he blamed her exhaustion on chronic poisoning and advised her not to go back to the same job. Then he referred her to his wife, a reflexologist, and she had started having the soles of her feet massaged weekly. She had come urgently to ask me to write a letter to her employers recommending a change of job so that she did not handle poisons any more. This came as a shock to me. I felt hurt that she did not give me any credit for her improvement, that she had so readily adopted such a simplistic and naive view of her illness, and that after all my efforts she had found a more satisfying kind of help from someone else. However, I was able to contain my hurt by reflecting that this is probably how parents feel when their children become strong enough to leave home. They have done a good job if the children feel confident and secure enough to look for people to love outside their immediate family. After a few moments of hesitation, I realised that I did not want to antagonise any agent that might be helpful to her. I expressed my scepticism about the cause of her symptoms, but as I knew that she did not like killing insects and animals I wrote the letter and gave it to her. I asked her to come again to tell me of her progress.

Two weeks later she told me for the first time since I had known her that she felt 100 per cent better.

Several things had happened to contribute to her well-being. First of all, she was praised by Mark's family for the good effect she was having on him by helping him to grow up. Rose had never been praised before and she lapped it up. Her boss at work agreed to redeploy her to a job that did not involve handling chemicals. Also, she was having hydrotherapy at the physiotherapy department for her body pains; massage and reflexology weekly, plus homoeopathic treatment. She was enthusiastic about reflexology. She found that massaging the soles of her feet made her relax all over. In fact, she was so enthusiastic that she decided to study reflexology herself and become a therapist. She had already enrolled in an intensive course.

Two weeks later she came to see me again, beaming and exuding well-being. Her clothes were smart and she looked younger and beautiful. I asked her about her progress and she launched into an excited and animated account of her reflexology treatment and her new training.

Suddenly there was a lot of purpose and meaning in her life. She explained how reflexology works and showed me the various areas of her feet on which parts of the body are represented. 'Perhaps I should treat you one of these days', she said. There was a genuine warm feeling between us. I laughed and replied that I would wait until she was qualified. Then I told her how pleased I was that she looked so much better.

Two weeks later she came back to tell me more about her progress. She had brought her books to show me, and with undiminished enthusiasm she said that in one of her courses she had met a chiropodist who taught her about the use of aromatic oils. She had started massaging her tummy in a clockwise motion with warm castor oil. Her bowels had become completely regular and so had her periods. She had cancelled the gynaecology appointment. I told her that she had never looked after herself so well before. 'Yes', she replied, 'I feel I am spoiling myself'. I told her that she had quite a lot of catching up to do. Then I asked her how things with Mark were. She grimaced. She said that he was a lot better. He still got his moods, but she would not let this affect her any more. I was pleased that her relationship to her body had changed so dramatically since I first met her: instead of tearing her skin to pieces, she was loving and caressing it with aromatic oils. This was a very impressive change that had to be supported and consolidated.

The Skin Envelope

Winnicott has said that 'chronic skin irritation emphasises the limiting membrane of the body and therefore of the personality. Behind this is the threat of depersonalisation and loss of body boundaries and of unthinkable anxiety which belongs to the reverse process of which he called integration' (Winnicott 1969).

Rose experienced two episodes of skin irritation. The first was related to her mother's illness and the second to her husband's unreliable behaviour towards their daughter. When Rose took her mother into her home, she relived the terrifying experience of her childhood, the beatings and threats of abandonment. She re-experienced the helplessness and the humiliation, the overwhelming anxiety and sense of worthlessness. One of the most primitive and terrifying fears is that of being dropped from the mother's lap, of being abandoned by the mother, of falling for ever and going to pieces. The effect of this fear is a disintegration of the personality. The anxiety is almost physical and unthinkable. The irritation of Rose's skin both defended her from and expressed this anxiety in a physical form.

Recognising her intense fear of abandonment made me adopt the holding attitude, and by inviting her to come and talk at regular intervals, I had caught her in her fall and provided the holding that she was missing at the time.

Rose could not experience anger at her mother despite her threatening behaviour, because any expression of anger would bring immediate retaliation and the fear of abandonment, and therefore of disintegration. My interpretation of her skin irritability has to be seen within the holding context. I was trying to put an unthinkable situation into words so that it could be thought about and elaborated. Rose's relationship to her mother was so disturbed that she had to defend herself by splitting the experience in two. The two dreams that Rose reported to me after the death of her mother express the essence of her conflict. In the first, she has to make her way through brambles. Suddenly she comes to the end of the brambles. There is a precipice and she falls. The fall caused a pressure in her chest and she woke up terrified. In this dream, falling symbolises the terror of losing the internal holding mother and therefore of disintegration. In the second dream Rose was looking for her daughter and could not find her; she was calling her but there was no response. Her husband told her that Rachel was asleep. Rose woke up in terror and went to check if Rachel was all right. Both dreams attempt to deal with the terror of losing the internal mother; the two aspects of the mother are dreamt separately.

The one who tears Rose's skin with her physical punishments is represented by the brambles, and the comforting mother by her daughter. It was impossible for Rose to think that she could be freed from one aspect of her relationship to her mother without at the same time losing the other.

Patients who had a faulty relationship with their mothers tend unconsciously to select partners with whom they can repeat the pathological relationship of their childhood. Their relationship to their bodies also recreates aspects of the maternal care system that handled their body during infancy and childhood.

Rose's relationship to her husband and her physical symptoms could be seen as a repetition of her faulty past relationship to her mother. However, three years passed before I found the right moment to interpret this to Rose, telling her that when her husband is in a foul mood, he becomes her angry mother and she becomes the frightened little girl; she loses her adulthood and therefore her self-esteem. This interpretation made her conscious of the repetition of her past into the present, and she became able to liberate herself from the compulsion to repeat the past. She was able instead to look for the mothering she always needed: the healing, tender, soothing touch of another woman.

As we have seen, Rose never gave me any credit for her improvement. Was it because she was afraid to tell me anything nice in the same way she never dared tell her mother? Or because she could not acknowledge her dependence? It seems that our relationship obeyed the pattern of splitting that she established earlier in her life. She split her therapist into a listening part which was me, and a touching, comforting, soothing and relaxing part. This was divided among several therapists – her homoeopath, the reflexologist, the aromatherapist, the physiotherapist and finally the aunt. When first confronted by this, I felt hurt and rejected. Perhaps this was her only way of expressing her anger and contempt. Had I retaliated with anger I would have fitted into her pattern of splitting the mother into two parts: a rejecting, punishing one and a comforting, soothing one. She would have gone to the reflexologist in defiance of me rather than with my blessing and we would both have been the poorer. This phase of her treatment lasted three years. During this time she attended the surgery eighty-two times, either on her own or with Rachel. Most of the sessions lasted five or ten minutes, with seven lasting twenty minutes. This was at the time when her distress was intense and I had invited her to come and see me weekly. There was never any question of termination. She continued to come regularly and our relationship benefited from the investment of so much psychotherapeutic work, although this was not formal psychotherapy: she was seen mostly on demand.

Her dreams provided me with an early understanding of her conflict, yet she took three years to arrive at the point where she could use an interpretation to gain insight. It would be presumptuous, however, to assume that it was only the accuracy of the interpretation that helped. As Rycroft has pointed out (1985), an interpretation, at least when it is given tentatively, conveys to the patient the feeling that the doctor had been listening attentively, has remembered what the patient has said and has been sufficiently interested to listen and remember and understand. By indicating the doctor's sustained interest in the patient, interpretation plays an important part in maintaining a trusting relationship that facilitates healing but which is not based entirely on transference. Caring for the patient's body, adapting to the patient's needs, showing concern and behaving reliably in the professional setting all constitute the holding environment within which an interpretation can become meaningful. General practice is potentially the ideal setting for treating psychosomatically ill patients. These patients find it difficult to depend on one therapist alone. Both Michael Balint and Donald Winnicott recognised this phenomenon and referred to it as 'collusion of anonymity' and 'scatter of therapeutic agents', respectively. Rose's need to split her therapist was influenced by her attachment to a cruel mother that made integration of the caring aspects of the mother with the mother's actual behaviour intolerable. Facing up to the hurt of realising that I was not the only therapist enabled me to understand and tolerate the splitting. I remained in the background as a facilitating influence, someone who could keep in mind the irreconcilable elements of her internal world. Eventually an opportunity for interpretation arose which made conscious some aspects of her relationsip to her husband which were responsible for maintaining her misery, and she became able to develop a more self-caring attitude. General practice allows patients like Rose to titrate their relationship with the doctor according to their tolerance and need. This approach contrasts with work in the same setting with psychoneurotic patients who may need formal intensive psychotherapy.

Rose is Afraid to Identify with Her Mother

Rose remained well for three years until she was fifty-three. One February, six years after we first met, she complained with a dramatic expression that she was not feeling well. She looked remote and absorbed in her suffering and she was sighing frequently. She said that her cheekbones and her gums were numb and that she had a pain in her left loin. She felt very hot and clammy that day.

Her frequent sighing and panting suggested that some of her symptoms might be related to fluctuations of carbon dioxide in her blood, as a consequence of irregular upper chest breathing leading to hyperventilation syndrome, and so I started asking in a systematic way for characteristic symptoms from other organ systems. To my amazement she denied any breathing difficulties despite the panting and sighing. She also denied feeling dizzy and light-headed, even though she felt faint on standing up. However, she admitted that her heart was racing, that she ached all over, that she had cramps in her calves and that her muscles twitched. She had headaches, blurred vision, and her toes felt tingly. She had a dry mouth, a sense of lump in the throat, a bloated abdomen and she also felt nauseous. She was sleeping poorly and was waking at 3 o'clock in the morning with a sense of fear and tightness in the chest.

At this point I looked at the problem list in her notes and, to my amazement, I realised that the following day was the fifth anniversary of her mother's death. My excitement on recognising the root of her problem got the better of me, and instead of proceeding in a systematic way I asked her prematurely whether she realised that the following day was the anniversary of her mother's death. Her tears welled up and overflowed. 'No', she said, 'I was not aware of that ... ' 'My symptoms are real', she protested. 'I am not imagining them.' I assured her that I did believe they were real and that they were caused by carbon dioxide deficiency, which was brought on by the way she breathed.

I asked her to lie down on the couch so that I could demonstrate to her a healthier way of breathing. I explained hyperventilation syndrome to her and taught her how to breathe with the diaphragm. She found it very difficult at first, but with some effort she succeeded and felt calmer and more relaxed. As we had run out of time I asked her to visit the following week for a twenty-minute appointment, in order to explore her feelings further and consolidate the diaphragmatic breathing.

When she came back a week later she was feeling a lot better, but she had not found the diaphragmatic breathing easy and was worried in case whatever was wrong with her breathing might interfere with the supply of oxygen to her brain and cause her to become demented like her mother. I reassured her that the symptoms were caused by lack of carbon dioxide rather than oxygen, and were reversible. I noted her fear of becoming like her mother and encouraged her to talk to me about it. She told me that she was so busy with her housework that she hardly had any time to be with her daughter, Rachel. It felt as if she was on a treadmill. She had to change and wash the curtains every week, do the ironing, dust and hoover every day, and so on. She did not dare leave it for a day because it would only pile up and the next day she would have to do double the work. I asked what her mother was like with housework and she said that she was at it all the time. She used to rail at people whose houses were not clean and would call them dirty, awful, with no values, and so on.

At the end of the consultation I reinforced the diaphragmatic breathing. She told me that she had never been aware of breathing with her upper chest before. I admitted that although she must have been hyperventilating for a long time this was the first time that it was obvious to me, and I invited her to come to see me once more, a week later, for a twenty-minute appointment.

This time, she told me that she had felt well enough to return to work, but that she was itching all over and 'it was driving her doolally'. I examined her and she did have red, itchy blotches on her thighs, in the small of her back and in her armpits. However, she did not remember having had a similar problem five years ago around the time of her mother's death, and she told me that she could not believe that all her symptoms were due to her mind.

I asked her whether she ever thought of her mother, and she replied that she did so all the time. She was afraid of becoming like her mother. The older she got, the more fastidious she became, like her mother, and the more she looked like her. Even her toes were becoming like her mother's. She was afraid that her mother was taking her over. I asked what particular aspect of her mother she dreaded most and she said that it was her cruelty, also losing her temper and losing her mind and becoming demented.

I reassured her that looking like her mother did not necessarily make her behave like her mother. How she behaved was her choice.

Even though I did not offer her any more appointments at the end of the third consultation, these sessions were the beginning of a new phase of her treatment. They marked the beginning of a new phase of physical treatment with a combination of relaxation exercises and breathing retraining. This new approach was the result of developing new skills for the management of hyperventilation syndrome which modulated her physical symptoms sufficiently to make searching for alternative treatments less pressing.

Rose Develops Cancer

Six years had passed since we first met in August 1987 and our relationship was about to enter its final stage. Two months after starting a new job as a security receptionist at a social services office, and a year before she died, Rose was assaulted on two separate occasions by clients at work. The first time she got friction burns on her fingers when an aggressive client yanked the telephone receiver violently from her hand, and the second time, a month later, another client slapped her on the face and dragged her across the floor by the right arm. She was frightened because she had read somewhere that you can get cancer from a knock and she began attending the surgery in urgent consultations without appointments, complaining of a multitude of symptoms relating not only to the pain of her injuries but also to hyperventilation.

I offered to see her once a week for a twenty-minute appointment in order to contain her distress. I planned to do this by allowing her to talk about her feelings and reducing the intensity of her physical symptoms by encouraging her to breathe with the diaphragm. During these sessions, as the initial numbness that followed the assaults receded, she began to cry and realised that the assaults had aroused all the helplessness and humiliation she had experienced as a child in the hands of her cruel mother who used to beat her black and blue 'for her own good', as she put it. Although she would go so far as to say that she got annoyed when she heard in the news about people abusing children, she felt no anger at her mother or her assailants. She could not understand why she was punished in this way.

One day, just before Christmas 1993, she came to the surgery without an appointment and complained in great distress of pain in the right hypochondrium. As this was a new symptom suggestive of gall bladder disease, I asked the surgical registrar to see her in Casualty as an emergency.

Two weeks later she came with a routine appointment, and as she began to tell me that the tests had shown metastatic liver cancer from an unknown primary, she burst into tears. I was stunned. It took me several minutes to comprehend the significance of what she was telling me and I felt a wave of sadness. With both hands I squeezed her left hand and told her how sorry I was to hear her news. She was very concerned about how Rachel would respond to the news of her illness. The mother of a friend had died recently from carcinoma of the breast and she was afraid to mention the word cancer in case Rachel thought that her mother would be taken away from her. Her husband, Mark, had had an affair and had left home, and Rose was essentially a single parent. She could not afford to die and leave Rachel a motherless child. She wanted to fight the cancer with all the means she possessed in the hope of living longer, at least until Rachel was a teenager so that she could see that she was properly taken care of. She asked me whether there was any hope that she would get rid of the cancer if she fought it. When I said that the only assurance I could give her was that whatever happened I would see her through it, she told me that she was lucky to have me as a doctor.

For the next three months she continued to come to the surgery at regular intervals to tell me about her preparations for chemotherapy and her attempts to communicate with Rachel who had began to complain of abdominal pains and to cry at the smallest provocation. Although Rose was initially reluctant to use the word cancer, the child psychiatrist to whom I had referred Rachel in anticipation of her bereavement, as well as the vicar and Auntie Doris, felt that being open about the diagnosis was the best policy. As Rose was leaving home to go into hospital to have an intravenous catheter positioned for the slow infusion of cytotoxic drugs, Rachel burst into tears. This was the first time she cried directly in response to what her mother did. Until then she was crying for other reasons, such as when her little dog jumped up and burst one of the two balloons she was holding, displacing the source of her distress.

One month after the beginning of chemotherapy and four months before she died, Rose developed severe diarrhoea and vomiting, became dehydrated and was admitted to hospital where I visited her a few days later. Her appearance had changed dramatically since I had last seen her. Her hair had fallen out and her face looked drawn and thin, but was lit by joy when she saw me. She told me that the vomiting made her so ill that she thought she was dying. She talked with disgust about the vile stuff that she brought up and decided that chemotherapy was not worth it if the quality of her remaining life was going to be so poor. Then she told me that her peace of mind was shattered because Mark, who had initially agreed to respect her wishes to have Rachel brought up by her nephew and his wife, had changed his mind and now wanted to take his daughter to his family somewhere in the North of England. Rose did not think that Mark had the right character to bring Rachel up because he relied on alcohol and addictive drugs to control his mood. She was determined to prevent this and asked whether I would be prepared to write a letter she could use in court, testifying to his unsuitability of character. Because I wanted to do anything I could to help her, and because I identified completely with her concern to protect Rachel from an unreliable and potentially abusive parent, I agreed without much critical thought.

Hope and Denial

A few days before Easter and two months before she died, Rose was discharged home. It was spring, the trees were beginning to bloom and her hope blossomed alongside the flowers. For the next eight weeks I visited her every Wednesday. I used to meet her in the sitting room where she reclined on a sofa in front of a large window overlooking the park. On the mantelpiece behind her, Rachel had arranged her soft toys in a row so that they would look after her mother while she was at school. Rose would take great care of her appearance. She would wear elegant, colourful, long dresses, and would sometimes cover her head in a white scarf that gave her an ethnic appearance and sometimes in colourful turbans that made her look like a Hollywood star. She was taking a number of drugs, including a large dose of oral morphine which made her want to sleep most of the time. But she felt hungry and enjoyed her food, and although she complained of drowsiness she thought that long hours of sleep helped her to conserve energy. I felt that she was probably having too much morphine and advised her to halve the dose. She felt so much more alert after this that she immediately stopped it altogether, but she began to experience withdrawal symptoms and we had to negotiate a dose that seemed acceptable. She decided that she did not want to take morphine because she felt that drowsiness interfered with her visualisation technique. At first she viewed her liver as a flat surface like a tray and the cancer as an egg on it, which the surgeon could cut out. However, when the specialist told her that the cancer cells were more like grains of sand on a carpet, she changed the imagery somewhat. The liver remained a flat surface but the egg now was surrounded by small yellow dots that she was pushing to the edge of the liver, until they fell into the bowel and were carried away. When she became constipated she worried that the evacuation of cancer cells had slowed down and she became eager to take laxatives.

Her friends and family rallied round and were very supportive. They would visit daily and do the cooking and housework. A neighbour offered her house for Rachel to have a party on her seventh birthday so that Rose was not disturbed. The local priest held the ceremony for Rachel's first communion at Rose's house so that she could be present. Rose was amazed at the grace of her friends' and neighbours' helpfulness. She was not used to such kindness. I reflected on the irony involved in the fact that the deficit of kindness, affection and tenderness that she suffered in childhood in the hands of her cruel mother was being made good towards the end of her life by the patience, concern, reliability and devotion of those involved in her terminal care.

During this period she had two dreams that puzzled her. She dreamt that she was fighting with Mark who had shiny, black, thick hair. She had grabbed him by the hair which was coming out in handfuls. He was telling her that she had to come and live with his family. Then she dreamt of her mother who had locked her in the sitting room: when she tried to get out, the key stuck and would not turn in the lock.

The second dream reminded her that when she was Rachel's age her mother used to punish her by locking her up in a big cupboard and leaving her in the dark where she felt scared and helpless. She was worried that Rachel might be abused too if she went to live with Mark's family. As she said this, her eyes filled with tears and she cried.

The most punishing aspect of her cancer was feeling sick and vomiting. Her face became distorted in disgust as she remembered the vile green stuff that she brought up. 'The slime ... the stench ... It was horrible, horrible.' The way she talked about this made me wonder whether in some way it represented the cancer and all the negative emotions that overwhelmed her, as if the vomiting was also, at some level, dramatising the ejection of badness. It was the colour and taste of bile that created the word 'melancholia'. But as this was neither the time nor the place for making interpretations I decided to keep all these thoughts to myself and, sounding as matter of fact as possible, I pointed out that it was the bile that gave her vomit such a bad taste.

Rose had embarked on another course of chemotherapy and continued blending hope with denial. She was determined to fight the cancer and felt that if she had a little more energy she would be fine. She was tired but comfortable, and a scan showed that the liver lesions had shrunk. Her improvement was so marked that she could go to West End shows with Rachel. After the seventh visit I suggested that perhaps it was not necessary to visit her every week. Although the necessity to visit someone at home who is capable of driving her own car and go to musicals is debatable, I had decided to continue visiting regularly in order to give Rose the experience of holding in this difficult time which comes from the attitude of reliability, concern and adaptation to the patient's needs.

The more healthy Rose appeared to be, the more sensitive Rachel became to her criticisms. She would burst into tears and accuse herself of not being able to do anything right, and sometimes she would even punch herself. We discussed the difficult situation Rachel was in and the contradictory feelings she must be experiencing. I wondered whether Rose's improvement made it safer for Rachel to experience some of the anger that she must have felt about her imminent abandonment by her mother. How could she possibly be angry with her ill mother? Punching herself could represent a turning of the anger against herself, or an atonement for her angry feelings, or both.

This idyllic time of unrealistic hope was coming to an end. Rose's liver began feeling uncomfortable, she began having pain at the tip of her right shoulder, she lost her appetite and started feeling sick. Despite chemotherapy, her cancer markers were soaring and her liver, which I could not feel eight weeks previously, had become palpable. Only a miracle would save her, and she decided to go to her birthplace in Ireland to visit a priest who had miraculous powers.

The Terminal Care

When we met again three weeks later, I was shocked by her cadaverous appearance. Her eyes had sunk in their sockets and her skin had darkened. Her hair had grown back, but it was thin and short and gave her a boyish appearance which reminded me of Joan of Arc. She told me that Rachel had been coming up to her and scrutinising her for a few moments, and when Rose asked what was wrong she would run away. She wondered whether she had become repulsive to her daughter. She had realised that she was not going to last long, but she was still hoping to live another four or five years, long enough to see Rachel become a teenager. I was moved to tears when I listened to her hopes, but her physical deterioration left me in no doubt that her survival was more likely to be a matter of four or five weeks rather than years.

Soon her oral medication was unable to control her pain and vomiting and the Macmillan team became involved, introducing a syringe drive to deliver a subcutaneous cocktail of diamorphine, tranquillisers and anti-emetics. They increased the dose every few days, and so her pain and fear were conquered at the price of profound tiredness and lethargy. As she became progressively more dependent, her older sister came to stay and look after them.

During one visit Rose told me that one of her many dreams was particularly vivid. She dreamt that she had stolen £4 from a booking office. She had £800 in her wallet, but she wanted to steal the £4 even though she knew she would be punished. When she stole them she went to the room next door where many people were crying and were asking her why she had to steal and be punished. We wondered whether the dream expressed her wish to steal a few more days, weeks, months or years on this earth. Rachel was telling Rose that she must not die before she had grandchildren. I asked Rose what her mother's attitude to stealing would have been, and both Rose and her sister shuddered. Rose remembered an occasion when she had picked up some discarded cards from a shop. When her mother found them in her satchel she had told her that when she came back from school she would be whipped. She had to go to school and think of the punishment all day. When she came back she was beaten with a strap. Both Rose and her sister then started telling stories about their mother's cruelty. She was a violent person and yet everybody else thought that she was the perfect housewife. She used to strip them naked and attack them with a strap. One day she pushed them out of the house and when in their desperation they decided to go to a neighbour, their mother pulled them in and beat them again. I commented that unfortunately you cannot choose your parents any more than you can choose to get cancer. It is the luck of the draw.

I felt very sad for Rose. A dream of my own two weeks before she died betrayed how much I resonated with the grief of her family. I dreamt of an emaciated woman who was sitting up and crying uncontrollably. Her partner said that under no circumstances must we give her alcohol, because she will not be able to control herself.

A few days later Rose complained of abdominal pain, and as I was about to examine her my nose became blocked and I felt I was suffocating. I wondered whether my sadness was getting the better of me and I had to practise diaphragmatic breathing to control my sense of suffocation. Rose noticed the difficulty, and after the examination was over she opened her hand bag and gave me a little paper bag with sweets for colds, saying that I would need it. Her sister found this amusing and said that we were treating each other. I felt that there was more truth in this statement than she imagined.

By providing the reliable, consistent, affectionate care that Rose had come to expect, I had become identified unconsciously with the loving and helpful mother that she had longed for; I felt that I carried the authority, influence and power of such a parent. Winnicott, in his brilliant paper 'Cure', has remarked that

the caring aspect of our professional work provides a setting for the application of principles that we learned at the beginning of our lives, when we were given goodenough care and cure so to speak in advance, the best kind of preventive medicine, by our good enough mothers and fathers. It is always a steadying thing to find that one's work links with entirely natural phenomena and with universals, and with what we expect to find in the best of poetry, philosophy and religion. (Winnicott 1986, p. 120)

In other words, I was doing for Rose what had been done for me at the beginning of my life, and as doing can be more effective than receiving in making up for past affective deprivations or misunderstandings, I felt that I was being helped as well.

I Identify with Rose

Two days before Rose died, her sister rang me at home, being very concerned because although Rose's death appeared to be imminent she was still hoping for a miracle and had neglected to secure a legal way to bar Mark from being Rachel's sole guardian. Her family were about to go to court to get an injunction to prevent Mark taking Rachel to his family and she asked me to write a report confirming that Mark's character was unsuitable for bringing up a young girl. Although I sensed the danger of writing such a damning report about a man who used to be my patient and of revealing medical information without his consent, my identification with Rose who wanted to protect her daughter from a potentially abusive parent was so strong that I agreed to go ahead and write that letter, ignoring the consequences.

When I visited Rose to deliver the letter I had expected to find her in a coma, so I was surprised to see her sitting up on the sofa looking drowsy. She looked at me inquisitively and when I told her that I had brought the letter she asked me to read it to her. By the time I finished she had become alert and looked excited. She thought I had not included enough damning detail in my letter and, gathering her syringe drive, she got up and staggered to her cupboard from where she took out a copy of her will. She read the part which stated emphatically that she did not want Mark to look after Rachel. She pointed to her will and said that when she died, it would not be worth the paper it was written on: my letter would be essential to support her wishes. Then she lit a cigarette and sat on the floor and cracked jokes and wanted to know what my first name was. When she found out that it was even more difficult to pronounce than my surname, she told me cheekily to keep it. Everybody laughed and the atmosphere became lighter.

Then she spoke of a vision she had had recently. She saw a bright, round, orange disc surrounded by small white dots. The disc gradually went further and further from her until it disappeared in the distance and she felt elated. I asked her whether it had a meaning and she told me that she visualised her liver as a round carpet, looking like a disc, and the cancer cells as grains of sand spread upon it. She imagined sweeping the carpet and throwing the sand down a tube that represented her bowel, from where it could be got rid of. It was obvious that in her vision the liver was not contaminated by cancer cells any more. In her imagination she had beaten cancer and she was elated.

I marvelled at her ability to maintain hope to the very end and felt very sad that she was slipping away.

Goodnight Rose

She died on a Saturday, and I visited as soon as her sister rang me. As I looked at the death certificate the Macmillan doctor had given the family and became aware of my mild rivalry with her, I reflected that I had always had to share Rose's care with other professionals, and this was probably just as well because I felt that I could not have tolerated the full force of her emotional needs by myself.

Rachel was being comforted in the arms of a friend. She had cried and wailed when her aunt had told her of her mother's death, but by the time I arrived she had regained her composure and was calm, looking at me with a quizzical expression. I told her how sorry I was that her mother died and that she must not be ashamed to cry. I followed her into her bedroom where she opened her diary and wrote: 'Mum has passed away.' Then she looked around and said how untidy her bedroom was. I did not know what to say and felt embarrassed. Her cousin came to join us and I suggested that all three of us played the squiggle game which would allow us to communicate in a soothing, comforting manner without having to say very much. Just before I left them playing together a few minutes later, I invited Rachel to come and see me at the surgery whenever she wanted. When she replied that she did not go anywhere by herself and that she did not even know how to pay the rent, I realised that perhaps she feared that now that her mother was dead she would have to do everything by herself. I tried to comfort her and tell her that her mum's loving family was going to look after her and do for her whatever mummy would have done, including bringing her to my surgery, should she wish.

It was time to go.

I went into Rose's room and with my right hand I made the sign of the cross above Rose's forehead, just as my mother used to do when she said goodnight before she turned off the light. Goodnight Rose. Goodbye Rose.

At the funeral a week later, Rachel did not display her distress. She remained very self-controlled throughout the service and I hoped that she would receive the right support to endure the grieving that she would have to do for the rest of her life.

CONCLUSION

The general practitioner who does not avoid engaging emotionally with his patients experiences the full force of their emotions with which he resonates. This experience can be very painful but it can be understood and the mental pain mitigated by having the emotional skills to process it cognitively and symbolically. However, the general practitioner remains vulnerable to becoming overidentified with his patients without realising it and acting in ways that, although beneficial to the patients, may bring the doctor into conflict with others. Whereas the code of practice for counsellors and psychotherapists considers it a breach of their ethical requirements to practise without regular supervision and support, in general practice this need is not given priority. Considering that a general practitioner looks after several very ill people at any one time, it becomes obvious that engaging emotionally with all of them in the absence of emotional support can become an intolerable burden. As more and more patients expect to have not only their physical diseases diagnosed and treated efficiently but also their emotional needs understood and responded to adaptively, a change in medical culture is required that will allow recognition of the emotional needs of doctors, too. A humane approach to the patients can be enhanced only within a climate of emotional understanding for all involved in their care.

15   FROM MEDICAL CARE TO SELF-CARE

THE PROBLEM OF SELF-CARE

When we do not take self-care for granted it is legitimate to ask, 'How do we learn to take care of ourselves?' How do we learn to comfort ourselves when we are distressed? To relax enough so that we can fall asleep and stay asleep? To manage our emotions adaptively? And to prevent emotions from overwhelming us? How do we learn to soothe ourselves and prevent the physiological aspects of our emotions from overstimulating us? To pay attention to our tiredness and rest appropriately? In short, how do we learn to become self-caring, self-soothing, self-solacing and self-regulatory?

The capacity for self-care depends on a number of related functions, such as the capacity to recognise emotions, to distinguish between them, to express them in verbal language and to modulate their arousal so that they can be experienced in various grades of intensity and therefore be tolerated better. All these depend on the capacity for reflective self-awareness and sensitive self-observation.

One of the common reasons that patients visit their general practitioners is that they are frightened by the unpleasant somatic sensations caused by the physiological arousal of their emotions and expect their doctor to make them better or at least to reassure them that they do not suffer from a dreaded disease. In attempting to understand these patients and respond constructively to their predicaments I have found Henry Krystal's ideas particularly helpful (Krystal 1988). He observed that psychosomatic and addictive patients cannot use their emotions as signals for themselves and have difficulty in managing their emotions because these are not experienced as their own creation but passively, as if coming from a significant other. Their definition of love is based on an addictive fantasy which says that if you love me, you will take care of me and make me feel good for ever. Since all the bad feelings are the responsibility of another, it is up to the other and not the patient to make him feel better. For example, Laura, the patient presented in this chapter, once asked me to make her better by the end of the week, in time for a wedding in Madrid.

These problems are compounded if patients are alexithymic because of the form taken by their emotional response. Attention is focused on the intense somatic sensations caused by the physiological arousal of vague and undifferentiated emotions, and the message contained in the cognitive aspect of their affects is ignored.

An associated problem, incapacity for reflective self-awareness, is also typical of alexithymia and interferes with the capacity to identify feelings as the appropriate response to self-evaluation. Such a deficiency in reflective self-awareness not only makes it impossible for such patients to utilise psychodynamic psychotherapy but also interferes with their ability to soothe and comfort themselves in an adaptive way.

WHY IS EMOTIONAL AWARENESS IMPORTANT?

Theoretical support for the importance of emotional awareness comes from disregulation theory which Schwartz summarises in the following way (Schwartz 1989).

All functioning systems are by definition self-regulating. If the various components of such a system are disrupted, or in exceptional cases disconnected, it will become disregulated. A disregulated system will show disordered behaviour that in extreme cases may be defined medically as disease. One psychological state that produces critical neuropsychological disconnection is disattention to essential negative feedback. Defence mechanisms, especially repression, denial, ignoring of emotional reality and disavowal, lead to lack of reflective self-awareness. This should promote demonstrable neuropsychological disconnection. According to disregulation theory, disattention should involve disconnection, create disregulation and promote disorder, which contributes to disease.

Conversely, self-attention to negative feedback, such as reflective self-awareness, should involve reconnection, create self-regulation and promote order (homoeostasis) which would contribute to ease or health.

Reflective self-awareness may have automatic self-regulatory, homoeostatic effects which increase the ability to engage in appropriate self-healing.

The disregulation theory underpins the practice of biofeedback which makes it possible to acquire control of parts of our body, which are normally controlled by the autonomic nervous system and therefore not accessible to volition, by paying attention to physiological processes with the help of electronic devices or simply self-observation.

Schwartz, for example, has demonstrated that patients who paid attention to their heart rate by feeling their pulse, and their respiration by feeling air come in and out of their nose, developed a slower heart rate and deeper and more regular respiration (Schwartz 1973).

From observations like these it is tempting to draw the simplistic conclusion that we can promote self-healing in all patients by drawing their attention to their physiological processes.

However, Schwartz and Krystal both refer to the important observation that in certain individuals self-monitoring during biofeedback can make them feel more anxious and distressed. Biofeedback therapists have reported a phenomenon that they call 'relaxation-induced anxiety' shown by some subjects practising relaxation. Schwartz explored this phenomenon with an experiment that compared the feelings of true low-anxiety subjects during a relaxation session with those of subjects who only appear calm because they repress anxiety. He found that whereas the first group experienced the relaxation as enjoyable and restful, the second group found it boring and unpleasant. He therefore suggested that if subjects who deal with their emotions by ignoring them suddenly become aware of their negative emotions during the relaxation session, they may find this unpleasant.

Although most studies of biofeedback have been made by behaviourists who pay little attention to the inner life of their patients there are some rare exceptions. Rickles is such a rarity in that he is also a psychoanalyst concerned not only with the patient's behaviour, but also with the psychic reality of the patient's mental representations and transferences to the biofeedback machine and the therapist. He has reported that some of his patients who were having psychoanalytic psychotherapy as well as biofeedback training abandoned biofeedback because they were frightened by the depressive feelings that emerged when they relaxed (Rickles 1981).

Krystal, who also used psychoanalysis to treat several patients who had undergone biofeedback training for psychosomatic conditions (such as intractable hypertension, very rapid heart rate, insomnia and headache), found that although most complied with the instructions of the psychologist and achieved some desirable results during the sessions, they nevertheless found it difficult to practise at home and to generalise their newly acquired skills to their everyday lives. Among the reasons for this failure, Krystal was particularly struck by the evidence of guilt and anxiety that all patients showed about gaining control over vital functions and over parts of themselves that they had assumed to be beyond their control.

Some were conscious of this feeling and expressed a fear that such a Promethean act on their part would be punished severely. Others dreaded that the acquisition of such powers might destroy them. Others showed indications of unconscious reactions in similar vein. Patients felt they were not allowed to exercise their volition on major parts of their bodies and that it was forbidden to take control over such functions as varying the depth, rate and pattern of respiration, lowering their heart rate and blood pressure and relaxing the muscles of their bodies and blood vessels. Krystal found that these feelings are universal and not limited to psychosomatic patients, in whom they are, however, more intense. He has come to the conclusion that this indicates an inhibition or emotional block to the exercise of potential function, rather than with peculiarities of the autonomic nervous system itself. Very often the inhibition includes all those parts of the body that are involved in an individual's affective responses.

WHAT LIES BEHIND THE INHIBITION OF SELF-CARE?

Krystal has come to the conclusion that behind this emotional block to the exercise of self-soothing and self-solace lies a distortion of the self and object representation. This means that the person perceives all good feelings as coming from the mother, so that to provide such sensations for oneself is to take over the mother's function. This usurpation of maternal privileges is the feared transgression against the natural order of things.

In this distortion, all the vital and affective parts of the body are attributed to the sphere of control of the mother, the 'object representation', and are excluded from the self-representation. The object representation is not recognised as our own creation because a barrier deprives it of the conscious recognition of selfhood. The question arises as to whether it is permissible for one to take charge of one's vital and affective functions and visibly and consciously carry out self-regulatory and self-caring functions. These distortions in self and object representation interfere with the gradual acquisition of self-soothing. They are more likely to occur when the mother–child relationship is not satisfactory. An atmosphere of love and trust is essential for the child to develop self-soothing capacities, from which evolve many other functions based on the freedom to solace oneself and create helpful images and ideas. Psychosomatic and drug-dependent patients are not free to take care of themselves, except by order of the transference, or under the influence of the placebo, or when the doctor gives them permission to do so. I suspect that this may partly explain why some of the patients who suffer from hyperventilation syndrome find it so difficult to benefit from breathing exercises and to change their breathing pattern from upper thoracic to diaphragmatic.

THE TYPE OF TRANSFERENCE RELEVANT TO INHIBITION OF SELF-CARE

The inhibition of self-caring is based not on the type of transference that psychoanalysts are accustomed to find in the treatment of neurotic patients, but on one derived from identification with the caretaking mother. Unlike neurotic inhibitions, it cannot be overcome by interpretation alone.

Many of the memories of the psychosomatic patient are affective, mostly pre-verbal, devoid of verbal or symbolic components. Psychic suffering at the pre-symbolic level is indistinguishable from physical suffering. This is the area of experience that Michael Balint called the 'basic fault'. The study of the difficulties encountered when trying to understand the emotional experience of these patients has given rise to the concept of alexithymia (see also Chapter 3). Because this deficit in the cognitive processing of emotions makes it virtually impossible for alexithymic patients to utilise psychodynamic psychotherapy, a preparatory phase of treatment is necessary in which the affective problem is attended to. I call this 'emotion coaching'. It is an educational process that helps the patient to identify certain somatic sensations as the physiological responses of affects, the cognitive aspects of which are either absent or isolated. After bringing these elements together the patient can start saying: 'I feel sad', or 'angry', or 'humiliated', instead of saying: 'I feel horrible', 'bad', 'anyhow', 'not myself'.

PROMOTING REFLECTIVE EMOTIONAL SELF-AWARENESS THROUGH INTEPRETATION ALONE IS NOT ENOUGH

Krystal has defined psychosomatic illness as an attempt to heal a lesion resulting from hyperactivity of the physiological component of an affect of the infantile variety; that is to say, undifferentiated and mostly somatic. The implication is that the doctor who engages in emotion coaching will also have to attend to the patient's bodily ailments which will have to be treated in their own right by physical or pharmacological means.

Emotion coaching, which involves the integration of the somatic with the cognitive aspects of an emotion and, ultimately, the integration of the self with the object representation, sounds easier than it actually is.

Patients who are not emotionally aware experience the integration of their self and object representation as exceedingly dangerous: coming anywhere close to such a possibility unleashes their defensiveness. For the ego to acknowledge unpleasant and threatening impulses, perceptions, ideas and emotions as belonging to itself is a way of owning all these things. This acknowledgement can be painful and hateful, but it means knowing as much of what is and was there as can be tolerated. This is a giant step toward attaining Identity, authenticity and the ability to love. The work of accepting what needs to be accepted and recognising that we are what we feel, requires effective grieving. To be able to mourn, however, one has to have available adult affects. These are precisely what alexithymic patients lack. The experience of undifferentiated, mostly somatic, unverbalised affect responses which are so painful and intense and threatening that we must ward them off by deadening ourselves or escaping into denial, can strangle the responses to grief and promote rage. Good affect tolerance is essential in order to carry out the process of mourning without it snowballing into a maladaptive state of depression.

The effective work in psychodynamic therapy is effective grieving, a process analogous to mourning by which one can give up attachment to infantile self-representation and the infantile view of oneself.

Krystal has found that many patients are angered by the idea of self-caring. They refuse to consider any renunciation of their wishes for concrete gratification of infantile sexual and aggressive needs, instantly, magically and simultaneously and they demand that someone else loves them and makes them feel perfectly well. The infantile view is one in which all feelings are the responsibility of the mother and it is up to the mother or her representatives, such as the doctor, to make the patient feel better. The healing principle of psychodynamic therapy consists in patients reclaiming their own minds, restoring conscious recognition of their selves, taking care of themselves and regulating their functions with conscious self-awareness.

However, when we try to understand the nature of psychic reality that makes it so difficult to lift repression from the maternal object representation so that it can be recognised as one's own creation, we are led to the core of the emotional problems represented by the infantile trauma. Many drug-dependent and psychosomatic patients have experienced infantile trauma and have to repress their rage and destructive wishes towards their maternal love object. By doing so they manage in fantasy to protect the love object from their magically empowered destruction and can assume that someone out there loves them and will take care of them.

Peter Sifneos, who coined the word 'alexithymia', used to advise psychotherapists to leave psychosomatic patients to physicians because real doctors get along better with them. This is not only because doctors do not try to uncover their deep secrets, but also because they are willing to continue to act as the caretaking parent who gives periodic permission to go on improving self-care for specified periods of time.

Although I never administered an alexithymia questionnaire to the patient I am going to describe below, and therefore I doubt whether she was truly alexithymic, she did complain with great intensity of a great number of somatic symptoms which can be understood as psychosomatic. In my work with her I ignored the advice of Sifneos in order to help the patient appreciate that some of her symptoms were an integral part of her emotions, which, like her dreams, were her own creations. It took a very long time and much patience, but finally my efforts were rewarded by a partial success. Laura gradually came to recognise that she was not the passive victim of invading alien forces that caused physical symptoms. She discovered that, to a certain degree, she herself was responsible for them and she learned to control them so that her emotions no longer overwhelmed her.

EXPERIENCING EMOTIONS AS AN ALIEN FORCE

Laura

Laura was forty-seven years old when she first came to see me in February 1988. She is a short, plump, Spanish woman who speaks fluent English with an attractive Spanish accent. Since she first registered in our practice in 1980 she has suffered from a variety of psychosomatic symptoms such as allergic swelling of the face, hives, hay fever, severe headaches, bouts of abdominal pain, recurrent attacks of diarrhoea and vomiting, dyspepsia, breathing difficulties, and generalised aches and pains. Lately she had started to fall occasionally and had developed a fear of leaving her flat.

At the start of our relationship she used to present her symptoms with an anguished expression and dramatise her suffering by wincing at every twinge of pain and rubbing the part of the body that hurt at the time. She would complain with extreme intensity, often beginning the consultation by saying that she was not better and the pains were killing her. I remember being filled with dismay at the beginning of every consultation when I realised that none of my conventional remedies worked.

As investigations and treatment of her physical complaints had given no result I decided that a different approach was essential. I asked her to make a double appointment – that is, one of twenty minutes – every time she came to see me so that we had time to talk. My aim was to give her the opportunity to explore her feelings and ideas and talk about them so that her physical symptoms would lose their intensity and would stop being the main form of communication between us.

Gradually I learned that Laura was the second youngest of sixteen children, and had lived alone with Sally, her seventeen-year-old daughter, since her divorce two years after Sally's birth. She described her husband as a 'Jekyll and Hyde' character. One day he told her a terrible secret and after that she did not let him touch her again. She felt that if she could share this secret with somebody she would not get any more headaches, but just the thought of it choked her and she did not want to talk about it.

She was almost crippled by her intolerance of anything smelly or dirty. What stopped her from leaving her flat was her repugnance at dirty, scruffy people who spit in the street. She was disgusted with sexual fluids and had to shower as soon as she and her husband had made love. Later, she was so disgusted with her daughter's dirty nappies that she started potty training her from the age of two months. She had always lived with her daughter in a close, mutually dependent relationship, but recently she seemed to feel increasingly threatened by Sally's developing independence and budding sexuality. She said that she could not keep up with her brilliant daughter and preferred the relationship she had had with her up to the age of fifteen. She would get furious with Sally for smoking or coming home tipsy after a few drinks with friends. After a row, she would develop a number of frightening symptoms which would intimidate Sally into submission. Sometimes she would have a fall after such a row. The clamour of her rage and the accompanying physical symptoms would protect her from experiencing any anxiety about her changing relationship to Sally, or from thinking about it in order to adapt to her new circumstances. From the day of her first appointment with me in February 1988 until February 1992, I saw her 100 times. Sessions from the beginning, the middle and the end of that period demonstrate her progress.

Laura developed severe back pain a few weeks after we first met and she stayed in bed for about a month. I treated her at home with analgesia and domiciliary physiotherapy. Sally had to do everything for her during this illness. Bath her, cook for her and when she became constipated she even gave her enemas. When Laura had recovered she started coming to the surgery regularly. One day she came to the surgery complaining of severe headaches. In our discussion it emerged that the downstairs neighbour made a lot of noise and when Laura complained, the neighbour swore at her. Laura became very annoyed, and when she was annoyed she worried and got a migraine. I asked what the worry was about. She said that she was worried that she might crack up in the same way that she had done at the council offices several years ago before she moved to her present address. She had gone to the council to complain about her neighbours, whom she described as 'blacks, Irish, madmen', who made a lot of noise and with one of whom she had had a fight. She went 'mad' in the housing office, screaming and shouting, overwhelmed with rage. I suggested that she had lost her head on that occasion, and that now the headache seemed to be an attempt to keep her head.

Laura's symptoms deteriorated. She missed the following appointment because she was too ill to get out of bed, and came to see me a week later in an agitated state of mind complaining of a multitude of physical symptoms. She had a chill from the top of her head to her toes as if somebody was 'walking on her grave', constant headaches, a tickling cough, a pain in her throat and breathlessness. She was breathless all the time but she would also wake up in the middle of the night gasping for air. She said that 'it' woke her up at 3 o'clock in the morning and she could not breathe. The air would not come out because there was a knot in her throat as if someone was strangling her. Sometimes she developed a heaviness on her chest and then she could not take a breath. It felt as if her chest had sunk into her tummy. Not surprisingly, she wanted me to examine her.

I was so impressed by her anxiety about the frightening and bizarre symptoms that I did not think about hyperventilation syndrome at the time. All I could find were some tender spots on her ribs. I told her that her symptoms were probably related to muscle tension due to her anxiety, and listened to her anger about the neighbour who was annoying her so much recently. Laura found it easier to talk of her rage with the neighbour than with her daughter, and considered the neighbour to be responsible for her state of mind.

When she said that 'it' woke her up at 3 o' clock in the morning, she was expressing her belief that she had no responsibility for her symptoms. She was the passive victim of something alien out there which attacked her in the middle of the night.

Krystal (1988) has pointed out that when affectivity is permanently blocked by long-lasting defences, the emotions are experienced as 'attacks'. During such attacks the affects may not be consciously recognised, as in the case of hyperventilation. This subjective experience causes the tendency for both doctors and patients to experience their emotions as if they were part of a physical illness.

My aim in treating Laura was to help her recognise her emotions as her own and her symptoms as somatic accompaniments of these emotions. Thinking about these emotions and expressing them in words could modify their intensity and make them a source of information about herself and her relationship to others.

This was not an easy task with Laura. Apart from her fear of being overwhelmed by the intensity of her emotions and going mad, there was also a fear that her magical powers would make the wish contained in the emotion come true. One day she told me she was trying hard not to make bad thoughts. She had the impression that she was psychic, that if she thought of something it would happen. 'Nothing good ever happens to me', she used to say. When her brother-in-law developed leukaemia she felt responsible and guilty. She remembered an argument they had had in Spain long ago, when she lost his dog and he told her off angrily. She was annoyed with him and she thought, 'Why don't you get lost like your dog?' Now she considered herself to be the cause of his illness.

About a year and a half after our first meeting Sally found a well paid executive job in an advertising company and, to celebrate her success, she went to Spain to visit her maternal grandmother. Laura developed severe back pain about a week before Sally left and colicky abdominal pains, diarrhoea and vomiting during Sally's absence. For these she made several requests for home visits. I felt dismayed that in spite of spending so much time with her during the previous year I had had so little impact on her neediness. Her symptoms did not improve after Sally's return. She complained of severe abdominal pains for which no drug was effective.

Sally now made an appointment with me to find out what was wrong with her mother. Laura had become afraid that she was suffering from a peptic ulcer and had asked me to refer her for a barium meal. Even though I knew empathically that her symptoms were related to her feelings about being abandoned by Sally during her trip to Spain, at some level I experienced her request for physical investigations as a vote of no-confidence. I felt that my authority was challenged, that it was my job to decide when physical investigations are needed. Her request implied that I was neglectful and this annoyed me. However, I was able to hold my anger and modulate it by reflecting on it with the help of earlier experience with psychosomatic patients (Zalidis 1991). This has confirmed Winnicott's view that their tendency to consult many therapists is a symptom of the split in personality organisation. There is little to be gained by forbidding this disposition. The patient will consult other therapists behind the doctor's back if there is a suspicion that the doctor disapproves or is expressing anger. Much can be gained if the doctor tolerates his own anger, stays in the background and maintains a unified view of the patient's progress. In relation to Laura, I could either have refused her request on the grounds that a similar test several years before had been normal, or given in to her request for a barium meal. Both options would have been dismissive, giving vent to my annoyance. On reflection the most helpful course of action would be to refer her to a consultant gastroenterologist. Apart from reassuring her, the referral would free me from the pressure to do something about her physical symptoms in order to concentrate on the psychotherapeutic management. Besides, as her symptoms were not improving, I was also beginning to consider a possible organic lesion.

I wrote to the consultant explaining the background of Laura's symptoms and personality, asking her to rule out organic pathology. Fortunately all the investigations were normal except for a raised eosinophil count (a particular type of white blood cell) which necessitated examination of her stool for ova and parasites. I remember with a certain vengeful glee the combination of amusement and horror on her face when she told me of the ordeal of having to put her stool in a pot and take it to the hospital for examination.

Very little had changed in her behaviour or her complaints since we had first met. The main gain was that by now she considered me to be her doctor and she always came to see me with a double appointment, something that was beginning to contain her distress within the practice. I would listen to her symptoms and then guide her to talk about whatever upset her most. Sometimes she was angry with her neighbour, but more often she talked about Sally. She would become furious if Sally came home drunk; jealous if she talked of her boyfriend, promotion and pay rise at work; tearful when she discussed her plans to work abroad, and annoyed because she spent all her money too easily without saving for the future. Very often she commented that their roles were reversed and Sally behaved towards her with the authority of a mother. One night she dreamt she was a cripple and was driving around in an electric wheelchair.

In November 1990 she developed sudden crippling back pain. The duty doctor had to visit her at home twice in order to assess her condition and treat her. She arranged for domiciliary physiotherapy and I visited three days later.

Laura was in bed and in a lot of pain and she greeted me with a barrage of complaints. 'The stupid tablets make me dopey ... the physiotherapist was no good ... her treatment was too short and ineffective.'

I asked whether she felt that Sally was caring enough and Laura wondered whether her pain had anything to do with her daughter. I asked how the pain had started. The day before the onset, Sally came home tipsy, giggling. Laura was furious. They had a violent row which lasted for three hours. At the height of the argument Laura slapped Sally and Sally slapped her back, breaking Laura's glasses. Sally stormed out of the flat and Laura spent all night sobbing on the floor. The following morning she went into the garden to cut some flowers to decorate her father's photograph. As she stretched her arms to cut the flowers she heard three cracks in her back and felt excruciating pain. She said that it was all Sally's fault and that she wanted to scare her into not drinking. Seeing her drunk reminded her of her husband. It was not lady-like. She behaved like a tart and Laura was afraid that any man could take advantage of her in that state. I commented that it would be an awful shame if she tried to control Sally with her back pain, but she took no notice. Laura said that there must be something wrong with her back and perhaps she needed an operation to put it right. I was worried about her trend towards invalidism: a cripple in a wheelchair totally dependent on Sally was a possible outcome to be prevented.

I visited her again two days later. Her pain was no better and she appeared to be in agony. Every movement caused excruciating pain and made her scream. I examined her and listened to her complaints about Sally who had left her alone for the day to go to a conference. She did, however, acknowledge that Sally did everything for her. She washed her, cooked for her, and if her constipation persisted she would give her an enema. I asked about enemas in childhood. She remembered her mother bringing her children breakfast in bed: first a cup of cappuccino and then a deep plate of boiled chestnuts to regulate their bowels. If she did not open her bowels within three days her mother would give her an enema. When Laura was about twelve, she told her mother to stop because she found it humiliating.

I visited again a week later and she complained bitterly of constipation. Sally had refused to give her an enema. She had rung the duty doctor at 3 o'clock in the morning in order to complain, but had not found his advice at all helpful. We talked again about her childhood in Spain. Her mother had to go back to work in a tomato factory after the birth of Laura's youngest sister, and one of her older sisters became the 'little mother' for her. She became the cleanest, tidiest child under the tutelage of that sister who was more fanatically clean than her own mother. She would run her fingers on surfaces that Laura had missed dusting and wipe the dusty finger on Laura's mouth. Her father was very much respected. According to Laura, he was 'a lovely man'. At dinner Laura would complain that her mother had given more food to her brothers and sisters. Father would ask her to hush and would give her a spoonful from his own plate. She missed him too much. She did not remember her mother ever kissing her, whereas her father did.

Her condition was not improving and I had to reassure the physiotherapist, who had anxiously rung me, that she was doing a good job.

When I visited again three days later Laura was in pain and full of complaints. Nobody was doing anything for her. She was angry with Sally who was not devoting herself completely to her mother's care. 'She could have given up her job for a few days', she said. 'Is her job more important than me? She does not care for me?' She was annoyed with Sally's excited chatter about the preparations for her company's Christmas party. She experienced this behaviour as a 'stab in the back', but a week later she felt a lot better. She could limp around the bed without much pain and was not complaining any more. During my visit, which had a social character, Sally came home with her new dress for the Christmas party. She was cheerful and excited and put it on to show us. I expressed my admiration but Laura said nothing and looked at it disapprovingly. When Sally went to the kitchen to make a cup of coffee, Laura said that she did not like the dress because it did not have any class. She went to her wardrobe and took out a black dress of her own that she had bought fifteen years ago to show me how much better class it was than Sally's. She had lost all interest in dressing up fifteen years ago, she said sadly.

The Turning Point

Then came a turning point. In January 1991, six weeks after the onset of her back pain, she was able to come to the surgery again. She looked somewhat amused and told me that she had dreamt she had sex with the Pope! I asked her for details. She had dreamt that she was in St Peter's Square. The Pope came up to her and held his hand out to her. He put his hand under her skirt and started fondling her. Gradually he made love to her and the whole thing was celestial, beautiful and refined. When Sally came into the room in the morning Laura felt so embarrassed. 'You will never believe what I have been dreaming', she told her. Sally laughed and laughed.

Since then Laura had been dreaming of the Pope every night. They did not make love any more but he cuddled her and it felt so good. In the dream, all his entourage treated her with respect, as though she was a member of his family. She was worried that she was going mad, for she was not even religious. She thought of writing to the Pope to ask him what he was doing in her dreams! I told her that as it was she who put him in to her dreams, it would be as if she put a picture of him in her sitting room and wrote to ask what he was doing in her sitting room. I reassured her that it was perfectly all right to have these dreams and asked her to come again in two weeks to talk more about them.

In retrospect it became clear from the ensuing guilt that this reassurance had not addressed the anxiety. When she arrived she started complaining of headaches and dryness of the skin on her nose. I asked whether she was going to waste her time instead of discussing her dreams as we had agreed. She looked at me craftily. 'I don't want to tell you my dreams, they are saucy.' Then she burst into laughter and said that a week previously she had dreamt of Patrick Swayze, the hunk who acted in the film *Dirty Dancing*. Then she told me of another dream with a different mood which she had dreamt after the Patrick Swayze dream. She was a Jesuit running through a forest. Hanging branches were whipping her face and she woke up with a feeling of suffocation, gasping for air. She often got this feeling of suffocation, she remarked. I asked, what would the Jesuits think about her dreams of having sex with the Pope? 'They would whip me, they would cut my head off', she said in alarm. I interpreted that in that case her dream expressed her guilt about the good times she had had in the previous dreams. When she asked what her dreams about the Pope meant, I suggested that the Pope stood for her father. She wanted her father to come and rescue her. Her back pain had started when she stretched her arms to cut some flowers to decorate his photograph. She marvelled, 'What a good memory you have!' She had never accepted her father's death. She had not dreamt at all for ten years, yet for the last two months she had been dreaming all the time. She also remembered dreams of being invited to tea by the Queen. She went to the Palace but was never given tea. When I told her that the Queen might stand for her mother she remembered how stingy her mother was, both with affection and money. Her father would not hesitate to spend money on her or encourage her to buy an extra pair of good shoes.

Laura's improvement was clearly signalled by her ability to remember her dreams. Although I did not make an interpretation, the Pope dreams expressed her wish for care and affection from me as well as from her father. Its sexualisation led to a sense of oedipal guilt expressed in her Jesuit dreams. This was so strong that it could not be contained within the dream but woke her up with a sense of suffocation. I wondered whether similar unconscious emotions and fantasies underlay the hyperventilation attacks that had woken her up several times at night in the past.

Laura continued to come to the surgery regularly but her physical symptoms had lost some of their urgency and now she could discuss her feelings. In November 1991 her mother became terminally ill with cirrhosis of the liver and her brother-in-law's leukaemia took a turn for the worse. She had to go to Spain to be with her mother, who died at the end of November.

Laura came to see me as soon as she returned. She told me how amazed she was with herself for finding the strength to overcome her disgust and nurse her mother. She had to feed her, wash her and wipe her bottom. She cried a lot when she died and now she felt empty.

In the middle of evening surgery, two weeks after her mother's death, I had an urgent request from Sally to visit her mother who was writhing in agony with severe abdominal pain. With a sense of exasperation I interrupted the surgery and visited her immediately. She was groaning with pain, twisting and turning in a world of her own. On examination she was tender all over. The slightest movement caused pain. I knew empathically that her pain was related to her feelings about her mother's death, but she was beyond words. I gave her an injection of pethidine and went back to the practice to continue my surgery. The injection did not work, and at 3 o'clock in the morning Sally called the duty doctor who admitted her to hospital under the surgical team.

In the morning Sally rang me at the practice. She was crying. Her uncle, her mother's brother-in-law, had just died of leukaemia and she was very worried about her mother. She wanted to know what was wrong with her. I explained that with such a degree of physical pain it was impossible to be sure that there was nothing seriously wrong going on in her mother's tummy. We would have to wait and see.

The same evening I visited Laura in hospital. She was drowsy from the analgesia and had an intravenous drip connected. The surgeons suspected intestinal obstruction. I sat by her bedside and we talked for half an hour. She remembered that something similar had happened to her when her brother died and she could not go to the funeral, and that her mother was complaining of abdominal pain while she was dying. Laura had had to go out of the room because she could not tolerate her moans. She felt so helpless. She had heard about her brother-in-law's death. She had known he was poorly but she did not expect him to die so soon. 'You have to bear so much pain Laura', I said. 'It is like becoming your mother and brother-in-law in one.' She groaned with pain. 'What can I do about it?'

Because I was worried that the surgeons might operate prematurely before giving her the benefit of the doubt, I rang the surgical registrar to inform him about Laura's personality and her tendency to respond to death events with severe pain. He had already noticed her capacity to dramatise and was interested in what I had to say. He was aware of an association between acute emotional crises and paralysis of the bowel.

Laura Begins to Own Her Emotions

The following day Laura's pain resolved and she was discharged. Four days later she went back to Spain for her brother-in-law's funeral. She suffered no more pain. When she returned she came to see me. She was sad and subdued and complained of feelings of emptiness and of shivering at night. She talked of her anger with her mother's helplessness. She was afraid that if she became paralysed Sally would have to do for her what Laura did for her mother, and she would not like this to happen. Life was so cruel and she felt so angry with it. I asked her whether it was possible that her abdominal pains had something to do with her anger. She looked at me in silence.

A month later she came back complaining of numbness in her hands and feet and a feeling of suffocation. She had not been able to take a deep enough breath for the last three weeks. She was also waking up at night, gasping for air. She wondered whether all these symptoms were due to her anxiety because Sally had gone to a conference in Greece, and with all the news about young girls being abducted and raped, she was worried. I explained hyperventilation syndrome to her and taught her diaphragmatic breathing.

When she came back three weeks later she said that she found the breathing exercises very helpful, but she still had a lot of headaches. We discussed her money worries and how angry she could be with Sally who spends money without a thought for the future. Then she paused and said that sometimes she thinks that she makes herself ill. I took note of this phrase. It represented a significant change from the phrase four years earlier that 'IT woke her up at night'.

She had begun to develop the capacity for reflective self-awareness and had stopped seeing herself as the passive victim of alien forces. She had begun to recognise that she owned her emotions and that her symptoms were their somatic accompaniment. It was crucial to this change that she had formed a relationship with me in which her long-standing depression, rage and denied sexuality could be acknowledged and contained, rather than expressed in symptoms and fights with her daughter and neighbours.

Conclusion

When I looked at Laura's medical notes after this period of intensive treatment, I realised that the number of consultations had fallen from thirty a year for 1989, 1990 and 1991 to fifteen for 1992. However, fifteen had been the average number before I adopted the emotion coaching attitude towards her. The dramatic change was not so much in the number of consultations as in their quality. There was no longer a sense of insatiable neediness and agitated demanding which made her come to the surgery without an appointment complaining of aches and pains and being oblivious to the disruption she caused to the doctor's work. She still attends frequently, but always makes a double appointment one or two weeks in advance, at which she discusses her feelings such as anger with her demanding invalid brother, or her apprehension about following her daughter to the US where Sally is tempted to live and work. She has been transformed from a patient whose urgent, incomprehensible, agitated complaints exasperated me into a person whose progress in life I follow with interest.

REFERENCES AND BIBLIOGRAPHY

Abramson, H. A. and Peshkin, M. M. (1961) 'Group psychotherapy of the parents of intractably asthmatic children'. *Journal of Children's Hospital Asthma Respiratory Institute* 1: 77–91.

Ader, R., Cohen, N. and Felten, D. (1995) 'Psychoneuroimmunology: interactions between the nervous system and the immune system'. *Lancet* 345: 99–103.

Alexander, F. (1950) *Psychosomatic Medicine*. Norton, New York.

Alexander, F. and French, T. M. (1946) *Psychoanalytic Therapy. Principles and application*. John Wiley and Sons, New York.

Ameisen, P. J. (1997) *Every Breath you take*. Landsdowne, Australia, Pty Ltd.

Anderson, C. D. (1981) 'Expression of affect and physiological response in psychosomatic patients'. *Journal of Psychosomatic Research* 25: 143–9.

Appleton, K., House, A. and Dowell, A. (1998) 'A survey of job satisfaction, sources of stress and psychological symptons among general practitioners'. *British Journal of General Practitioners*; 48: 1059–63.

Balint, M. (1957) *The Doctor, his Patient and the Illness*. Pitman Medical, London.

Balint, M. (1968) *The Basic Fault*. Tavistock Publications, London.

Balint, M. and Balint, E. (1961). *Psychotherapeutic Techniques in Medicine*. Tavistock Publications, London.

Balint, E. and Norell, J. S. (eds) (1973) *Six Minutes for the Patient. Interactions in general practice consultations*. Tavistock Publications. London.

Balkanyi, C. (1964) 'On verbalisation'. *International Journal of Psychoanalysis* 45 (part 1): pp 64–74.

Bartrop, R. W., Luckhurst, E. K. L. and Penny, R. (1977) 'Depressed lymphocyte function after bereavement'. *Lancet* 2: 834–6.

Basch, M. F. (1976) 'The concept of affect: a re-examination'. *Journal of the American Psychoanalytic Association* 24: 759–77.

Basch, M. F. (1988) *Understanding Psychotherapy. The science behind the art*. Basic Books, New York.

Bass, C. M. (1989) 'Functional cardiorespiratory syndromes'. in C. Bass (ed.) *Somatisation: Physical symptoms and psychological illness*. Blackwell, London.

Beck, A. T. Ward, C., Mandelson, M. et al. (1961) 'An inventory for measuring depression'. *Archives of General Psychiatry* 4: 561–71.

Berry, D. S. and Pennebaker, J. W. (1993) 'Nonverbal and verbal emotional expression and health'. *Psychotherapy and Psychosomatics* 59: 11–19.

Bettelheim, B. and Rosenfeld, A. (1993) *The art of the obvious. Developing insight for psychotherapy and everyday life*. Thames and Hudson Ltd, London.

Bollas, C. (1987) *The Shadow of the Object. Psychoanalysis of the unknown thought*. Columbia University Press, New York.

Bowlby, J. (1990) *Charles Darwin. A new biography*. Hutchison Publications, London.

Bowler, S., Green, A. and Mitchell, C. (1998) Buteyko breathing technique in asthma. *Medical Journal of Australia*: 169: 575–8.

Bradley, D. (1992) *Hyperventilation Syndrome: A handbook for sufferers*. Celestial Arts.

Breuer, J. and Freud, S. (1893). 'On the psychical mechanism of hysterical phenomena', in J. Strachey (ed.) *The Standard Edition of the Complete Works of Sigmund Freud.* Hogarth Press, London, 1958, vol. 2, pp. 3–17.

Brody, H. (1987) *Stories of Sickness.* Yale University Press, New Haven and London.

Brody, H. (1994) 'My story is broken; can you help me fix it? Medical ethics and the joint construction of narrative'. *Literature and Medicine.*13 (1): 79–92.

Brook, A. (1995) 'The Eye and I: psychological aspects of disorders of the eye'. *Journal of the Balint Society* 23: 13–16.

Brook, A., Dowling, M. B., Pollard, J. C., Bleasdale, M. B., Hopkins, J. H. S. and Stroud, A. R. (1966) 'Emotional problems in general practice'. *Journal of the College of General Practitioners* 11 (184): 185–94.

Brook, A., Elder, A. and Zalidis, S. (1998) 'Psychological aspects of eye disorders'. *Journal of the Royal Society of Medicine* 91: 270–2.

Brook, A. and Temperley, J. (1976) 'The contribution of a psychotherapist to general practice'. *Journal of the Royal College of General Practitioners* 26: 86–94.

Brook, A. and Zalidis, S. (1999) 'Blepharitis and grieving'. *Psychotherapy Review* 1(1): 23–5.

Brown, G. W. and Harris, T. (1978) *Social Origins of Depression.* Tavistock Publications, London.

Brown, G. W. and Harris, T. (1981) *Life Events and Illness.* Unwin Hyman, London, Boston, Sydney, Wellington.

Bruch, H. (1979) *The Golden Cage. The enigma of anorexia nervosa.* Vintage Books, New York.

Buckroyd, J. (1994) *Eating Your Heart Out. Understanding and overcoming eating disorders,* Optima, London.

Burton, C. D. (1993) 'Hyperventilation in patients with recurrent functional symptoms'. *British Journal of General Practice* 43: 422–5.

Bynner, W. (1943) *Selected Poems,* ed. R. Hunt. Alfred Knopf, New York.

Chada, D. (2000) 'Discrimination rife against mental health patients'. *British Medical Journal* 320: 1163.

Chekhov, A. (1886) *Early Stories,* trans. P. Miles and H. Pitcher. Oxford University Press, 1984, Oxford, New York.

Cluff, R. A. (1984) 'Chronic hyperventilation and its treatment by physiotherapy: Discussion paper'. *Journal of the Royal Society of Medicine* 77: 855–61.

Cornelius, R. R. (1996) *The science of Emotion. Research and tradition in the psychology of emotion.* Prentice Hall, New Jersey.

Damasio, A. R. (1996) *Descartes' Error. Emotion, reason, and the human brain.* Papermac, London.

Damasio, A. R. (1999) *The Feeling of What Happens. Body, emotion and the making of consciousness.* Heinemann, London.

Darwin, C. (1872) *The Expression of the Emotions in Man and Animals.* University of Chicago Press, Illinois, 1965.

De Botton, A. (1997) *How Proust can Change your Life.* Picador Macmillan, London and Oxford.

Deutsch, F. (1953) 'Basic psychoanalytic principles in psychosomatic medicine'. *Acta Therapeutica* 1: 102–11.

Deutsch, F. (1959) *On the Mysterious Leap from the Mind to the Body. A study of the theory of conversion.* International Universities Press, New York.

Deutsch, H. (1937) 'Absence of grief'. *Psychoanalytic Quarterly* 6:12–22.

Dicks, J., Jones, N. and Kinsman, R. (1977) 'Panic fear: a personality dimension related to intractability in asthma'. *Psychosomatic Medicine,* 39(2): 120–6.

Dodge, J. A. (1970) 'Production of duodenal ulcers and hypertrophic pyloric stenosis by administration of pentagastrin to pregnant and newborn dogs'. *Nature* 215: 284–5.

Dodge, J. A. (1972) 'Psychosomatic aspects of infantile pyloric stenosis'. *Journal of Psychosomatic Research* 16: 1–5.

Dodge, J. A. (1975) 'Infantile hypertrophic pyloric stenosis in Belfast, 1957–1969'. *Archives of Diseases of Childhood* 50: 171–8.

Dodge, J. A. and Karem, A. A. (1976) 'Induction of pyloric hypertrophy by pentagastrin'. *Gut* 17: 280–4.

Elder, A. and Samuel, O. (eds) (1987) *While I'm Here, Doctor. A study of the doctor–patient relationship.* Tavistock Publications, London.

Engel, G. L. and Schmale, A. H. (1967) 'Psychoanalytic theory of somatic disorder: conversion, specificity and the disease onset situation'. *Journal of the American Psychoanalytic Association* 15: 344–65.

Erikson, E. (1931) 'The fate of the drives in school compositions', in S. Sclein (ed.) *A Way of Looking at Things. Selected papers from 1930 to 1980.* Norton and Company, New York, London, 1987.

Evans, D. W. and Lum, L. (1981) 'Hyperventilation as a cause of chest pain mimicking angina'. *Practical Cardiology* 7(7): 131–9.

Fenichel, O. (1945) 'Nature and classification of the so-called psychosomatic phenomena'. *Psychoanalytic Quarterly* 14: 287–93.

Fitzgerald, R. G. (1970) 'Reactions to blindness: an exploratory study of adults with recent sight loss'. *Archives of General Psychiatry* 22: 370–9.

Freedman, M. B. and Sweet, B. S. (1954) 'Some specific features of group psychotherapy and their implication for selection of patients'. *International Journal of Group Psychotherapy* 4: 355–68.

Freeman, L. J. and Nixon, P. G. F. (1985) 'Chest pain and the hyperventilation syndrome: some aetiological considerations'. *Postgraduate Medical Journal* 61: 957–61.

Freud, S. (1905) 'Psychical (or mental) treatment'. *Collected Works.* Hogarth Press, London, vol. 7.

Freud S. (1917) 'Mourning and melancholia'. *Collected Works.* Hogarth Press, London, vol. 14.

Furman, R. A.(1978) 'Some developmental aspects of the verbalisation of affects'. *Psychoanalytic Study of the Child* 33: 187–212.

Galer, B. S. and Portenoy, R. K. (1991) 'Acute herpetic and postherpetic neuralgia: clinical features and management'. *Mount Sinai Journal of Medicine* 58(3): 257–66.

Gardner, H. (1983) *Frames of Mind. The theory of multiple intelligences.* Basic Books, New York.

Gardner, W. N. and Bass, C. (1989) 'Hyperventilation in clinical practice'. *British Journal of Hospital Medicine* 41: 73–81.

Garrow, J. S. (1988) *Obesity and Related Diseases.* Churchill Livingstone, Edinburgh.

Goleman, D. (1995) *Emotional Intelligence. Why it can matter more than IQ.* Bantam Books, New York, Toronto, London, Sydney, Auckland.

Gottman, J. (1997) *The Heart of Parenting. How to raise an emotionally intelligent child.* Bloomsbury, London.

Groddeck, G. (1977) *The Meaning of Illness. Selected psychoanalytic writings.* Hogarth Press, London.

Groen, J. J. and Pelser, H. E. (1960) 'Experiences and results of group psychotherapy in patients with bronchial asthma'. *Journal of Psychosomatic Research* 4: 191–205.

Halton, W. (1995) 'Institutional stress on providers in health and education'. *Psychodynamic Counselling* 1: 187–98.

Hayman, R. (1990) *Proust.* Minerva, London.

Heath, R. B. and Kangro, H. O. (1990) 'Varicella zoster', in A. J. Zuckerman and J. E. Banatvalla (eds) *Principles and Practice of Clinical Virology.* John Wiley and Sons Ltd.

Hennezel, M. De (1997) *Intimate Death. How the dying teach us to live.* Warner Books, London.

Hofer, M. A. (1983) 'The mother–infant interaction as a regulator of infant physiology and behaviour', in L. Rosenblum and H. Moltz (eds) *Symbiosis in Parents – Offspring Interactions.* Plenum, New York.

Holmes, T. H. and Rahe, R. H. (1967) 'The social readjustment rating scale'. *Journal of Psychosomatic Research* 11: 213–18.

Horowitz, M. J. (1988) *Introduction to Psychodynamics. A new synthesis*. Routledge, London.

Inman, W. S. (1946) 'Styes, barley and wedding rings'. *British Journal of Medical Psychology* 20: 331–8.

Inman, W. S. (1964) *Styes and Wedding Rings. Collected papers*. Churchill Livingstone, Edinburgh, London.

Jacobson, J. G. (1994) 'Signal affects and our psychoanalytic confusion of tongues'. *Journal of the American Psychoanalytic Association* 42: 15–42.

Jones, C. M. (1938) *Digestive Tract Pain: Diagnosis and treatment; experimental observations*. Macmillan, New York.

Kestenberg, J. S. (1978) 'Transensus, outgoingness and Winnicott's intermediate zone', in S. A. Grolnick, L. Baskin and W. Muestenberger (eds) *Between Reality and Fantasy: Transitional objects and phenomena*. Jason Aronson, New York.

Knapp, P. (1989) 'Psychosomatic aspects of bronchial asthma: a review', in S. Cheren (ed.) *Psychosomatic Medicine. Theory, physiology, and practice*. International Universities Press, Madison, CT.

Krystal, H. (1988) *Integration and Self-Healing. Affect, trauma, alexithymia*. Analytic Press, New Jersey.

Kübler-Ross, E. (1969) *On death and dying*. Macmilllan Publishing. Co. Inc., New York.

Lancaster, T. Silagy, C. and Gray, S. (1995) 'Primary care management of acute herpes zoster: systematic review of evidence from randomized control trials'. *British Medical Journal* 45: 39–45.

Lane, J, D. and Storr, A. (1981) *Asthma. The facts*. Oxford University Press, Oxford, New York, Toronto.

Lane, R. D. and Schwartz, G. E. (1987) 'Levels of emotional awareness. A cognitive developmental theory and its application to psychopathology'. *American Journal of Psychiatry* 144: 133–43.

Langewitz, W., Ruddel, H. and Schachinger, H. (1994) 'Reduced parasympathetic cardiac control in patients with hypertension at rest and under mental stress'. *American Heart Journal* 127: 122–8.

Lask, A. (1966) *Asthma, Attitude and Milieu*. Tavistock Publications, London.

Lazarus, H. R. and Kostan, J. J. (1969) 'Psychogenic hyperventilation and death anxiety'. *Psychosomatics* 10: 14–22.

Le Doux, J. (1998) *The Emotional Brain*. Weidenfield and Nicolson, London.

Liebman, R., Minuchin, S. and Baker, L. (1974) 'The use of structural family therapy in the treatment of intractable asthma'. *American Journal of Psychiatry* 131: 535–40.

Lofgren, J. B. A. (1961) 'A case of bronchial asthma with unusual dynamic factors treated by psychotherapy and psychoanalysis'. *International Journal of Psycho-Analysis* 42: 414–43.

Lum, L. C.(1976) 'The syndrome of habitual chronic hyperventilation', in O. W. Hill (ed.) *Modern Trends in Psychosomatic Medicine* vol. 3. Butterworths, London.

Lum, L. C. (1987) 'Hyperventilation syndromes in medicine and psychiatry. A review'. *Journal of the Royal Society of Medicine* 80: 229–31.

Luparello, T. J., Lyons, H. A., Bleecker, E. R. and McFadden, E. R. Jr (1968) 'Influence of suggestion on airway reactivity in asthmatic subjects'. *Psychosomatic Medicine* 30: 819–25.

McDougall, J. (1980a) *Plea for a Measure of Abnormality*. International Universities Press, New York.

McDougall, J. (1980b) 'The antianalysand in analysis', in S. Lebovici and D. Wildocher (eds) *Psychoanalysis in France*. International Universities Press, New York.

Maclean, P. D. (1949) 'Psychosomatic disease and the visceral brain. Recent developments bearing on the Papez theory of emotion'. *Psychosomatic Medicine* 11: 338–53.

McWhinney, I. R. (1998a) 'Core values in a changing world', in M. Pringle (ed.) *Primary Care: Core values*. BMJ Books, London.

McWhinney, I. R. (1998b) 'Core values in a changing world'. *British Medical Journal* 316: 1807–9.

Magarian, G. (1982) 'Hyperventilation syndromes: infrequently recognised common expressions of anxiety and stress'. *Medicine* 61: 219–36.

Martin, P. (1997) *The Sickening Mind. Brain, behaviour, immunity and disease*. HarperCollins, London.

Marty, P. et de M'Uzan, M. (1963) 'La pensée opératoire'. *Revue Française Psychoanalyse* 27 (suppl.): 1345–56.

Maudsley, H. (1868) *The Physiology and Pathology of Mind*.

Marris, P. (1982) 'Attachment and society', in M. Parkes and H. Stevenson (eds) *The Place of Attachment in Human Behaviour*. Basic Books, London.

Melzack, P. and Wall, P. D. (1996) *The Challenge of Pain*. Penguin Books, London.

Meneker, E. (1982) *Otto Rank. A rediscovered legacy*. Columbia University Press, New York.

Metzner, A. (1983) 'Hypertrophic pyloric stenosis: an adaptive crisis in the mother–infant relationship'. Unpublished dissertation.

Miller, W. I. (1997) *The Anatomy of Disgust*. Harvard University Press, Cambridge, MA, and London.

Minuchin, S., Rosman, B. and Baker, L. (1978) *Psychosomatic Families. Anorexia nervosa in context*. Harvard University Press, Cambridge, MA and London.

Nathanson, D. L. (1992) *Shame and Pride. Affect sex and the birth of the self*. Norton, New York, London.

Nesse, R. and Williams, G. (1997) 'Are mental disorders diseases?', In S. Baron Cohen (ed.) *The Maladapted Mind. Classic readings in evolutionary psychopathology*. Psychology Press Publishers, UK.

Nisbett, R. E. (1972) 'Hunger, obesity and the ventromedial hypothalamus'. *Psychology Review* 79: 433–53.

Nixon, P. G. F. (1994) 'Breathing: physiological reasons for loss of self control', in J. G. Carlson, A. R. Seifert and N. Birbaumer (eds) *Clinical Applied Psychophysiology*. Plenum, New York.

Odent, M. (1999) *The Scientification of Love*. Free Association Books, London.

O'Dowd, T. C. (1988) 'Five years of heartsink patients in general practice'. *British Medical Journal*, 297: 528–30.

Pally, R. (1998) 'Emotional processing: the mind–body connection'. *International Journal of Psycho-Analysis* 79: 349–62.

Paulley, J. W. (1990) 'Hyperventilation'. *Recent Progress in Medicine* 81(9): 594–600.

Paulley, J. W. and Pelser, H. E.(1989) *Psychological Managements for Psychosomatic Disorders*. Springer-Verlag, Berlin, Heidelberg, New York, London, Paris, Tokyo, Hong Kong.

Pearson, R. (1990) *Asthma. Management in primary care*. Radcliffe Medical Press, Oxford.

Pennebaker, J. W. (1985) 'Traumatic experience and psychosomatic disease: exploring the roles of behavioural inhibition, obsession, and confiding'. *Canadian Psychology* 26: 82–95.

Pennebaker, J. W. and Susman J. R. (1988) 'Disclosure of traumas and psychosomatic processes'. *Social Science and Medicine* 26: 327–32.

Pfeffer, J. M. (1978) 'The aetiology of hyperventilation syndrome'. *Psychotherapy and Psychosomatics* 30: 47–55.

Phillips, M. L., Senior, C., Fahy, T. and David, S. A. (1998) 'Disgust – the forgotten emotion in psychiatry'. *British Journal of Psychiatry* 172: 373–5.

Plato. *The Republic*. Trans. D. Lee. Penguin Classics (1987).

Platt, W. F. (1995) *Conversation Repair. Case studies in doctor–patient communication*. Little, Brown and Co, Boston, New York, Toronto, London.

Pollock, G. H. (1989) *The Mourning Liberation Process*. International Universities Press, Madison, CT.

Rice, R. L. (1950) 'Symptom patterns of the hyperventilation syndrome'. *American Journal of Medicine* 8: 691–700.

Rickles, W. H (1981) 'Biofeedback therapy and transitional phenomena'. *Psychiatric Annals* 11: 86–93.

Ruesch, J. (1948) 'The infantile personality'. *Psychosomatic Medicine* 10: 134–44.

Rycroft, C. (1985) 'What analysts say to their patients', in *Psychoanalysis and Beyond*. Chatto and Windus/Hogarth Press, London.

Salinsky, J. (1999) 'Hanging by a thread: the history of Balint in Britain 1972–1999', *Journal of the Balint Society* 27: 16–20.

Salinsky, J. and Sackin, P. (2000) *What are You Feeling, Doctor? Identifying and avoiding defensive patterns in the consultation*. Radcliffe Medical Press Ltd, London.

Salovey, P., Hsee, C. K. and Mayer, J. (1993) 'Emotional Intelligence and the self-regulation of affect', in D. M. Wegner and J. W. Pennebaker (eds) *Handbook of Mental Control*. Prentice Hall, Englewood Cliffs, NJ, pp. 258–77.

Sartre, J.-P. (1948) *The Emotions: Outline of a theory*. Philosophical Library, New York.

Schmader, K. et al. (1990) 'Are stressful life events risk factors for herpes zoster?' *Journal of the American Geriatric Society*. 38: 1188–94.

Schwartz, G. E. (1973) 'Biofeedback as therapy: some theoretical and practical issues'. *American Psychology* (August): 666–73.

Schwartz, G. E. (1989) 'Disregulation theory and disease: toward a general model for psychosomatic medicine', in S. Cheren (ed.) *Psychosomatic Medicine. Theory, physiology, and practice*. International Universities Press, Madison, CT.

Shoenberg, P. (1992) 'The student psychotherapy scheme at the University College and Middlesex School of Medicine: its role in helping medical students to learn about the doctor–patient relationship'. *Journal of the Balint Society* 20: 10–14.

Sifneos, P. E. (1973) 'The prevalence of alexithymic characteristics in psychosomatic patients'. *Psychotherapy and Psychosomatics* 22: 255–62.

Smith, R. (2000) 'Hamster health care'. *British Medical Journal* 321:1541.

Sperling, M. (1963) 'A psychoanalytic study of bronchial asthma in children', in H. I. Schneer (ed.) *The Asthmatic Child*. Harper and Row, New York.

Spezzano, L. (1993) *Affect in Psychoanalysis. A clinical synthesis*. The Analytic Press, Hillsdale, NJ, London.

Spiegel, D. et al. (1989) 'Effect of psychosocial treatment on survival of patients with metastatic breast cancer'. *Lancet* 8668: ii.

Sternberg, M. E. and Gold, W. P.(1997). 'The mind–body interaction in disease'. *Scientific American. Mysteries of the mind* (special issue): 8–15.

Stewart, M., Brown, J. B., Weston, W. W., McWhinney, I. R., McWilliam, C. L. and Freeman, T. R. (1995) *Patient-Centred Medicine: Transforming the clinical method*. Sage Publications, Thousand Oaks, London, New Delhi.

Stoller, R. (1985) *Observing the Erotic Imagination*. Yale University Press, New Haven and London.

Swanson, D. W. (1984) 'Chronic pain as a third pathologic emotion'. *American Journal of Psychiatry*. 141: 210–14.

Taylor, G. J. (1976) 'Alexithymia and the countertransference'. *Psychotherapy and Psychosomatics* 28: 141–7.

Taylor, G. J. (1987) *Psychosomatic Medicine and Contemporary Psychoanalysis*. International Universities Press, Madison, CT.

Taylor, G. J. (1994). 'The alexithymia construct: conceptualisation, validation, and relationship with basic dimensions of personality'. *New Trends in Experimental and Clinical Psychiatry* X(2): 61–74.

Taylor, G. J. (1995) 'Psychoanalysis and empirical research: the example of patients who lack psychological mindedness'. *Journal of the American Academy of Psychoanalysis* 23(2): 263–81.

Taylor, G. J. (2000) 'Recent developments in alexithymia theory and research'. *Canadian Journal of Psychiatry*, 45: 134–42.

Taylor, G. J and Bagby, M. R. (1999) 'An overview of the alexithymia construct', in R. Bar-On and J. D. A. Parker (eds) *Handbook of Emotional Intelligence*. Jossey-Bass, San Francisco.

Taylor, G. J. Bagby, M. P. and Parker, J. D. A. (1997) *Disorders of Affect Regulation. Alexithymia in medical and psychiatric illness*. Cambridge University Press, Cambridge.

Temoshok, L. et al. (1985) 'The relationship of psychosocial factors to prognostic indicators in cutaneous malignant melanoma'. *Journal of Psychosomatic Research* 29(2): 139–53.

Thomas, M., McKinley, R. K., Freeman, E. and Foy, C. (2001) 'Prevalence of dysfunctional breathing in patients treated for asthma in primary care: cross sectional survey'. *British Medical Journal* 7294: 1098–1100.

Tomkins, S. S. (1962) *Affect, Imagery and Consciousness*. Vol. 1. *The Positive Affects*. Springer Publishing, New York.

Tomkins, S. S. (1963) *Affect, Imagery and Consciousness*. Vol. 2. *The Negative Affects*. Springer Publishing, New York, Tavistock Publications, London.

Tomkins, S. S. (1991) *Affect, Imagery and Consciousness*. Vol. 3. *The Negative Affects. Anger and Fear*. Springer Publishing, New York.

Tomkins, S. S.(1992) *Affect, Imagery and consciousness*. Vol. 4. *Cognition*. Springer Publishing, New York.

Vaillant, E. G. (1993) *The Wisdom of the Ego*. Harvard University Press, Cambridge, MA, London.

Vrana, S. R., Guthbert, B. N. and Lang, P. J. (1986) 'Fear, imagery, and text processing'. *Psychophysiology*, 23: 247–53.

Wadden, T. and Stunkard, A. (1989) 'Obesity: Etiology and treatment of a major medical problem', in S. Cheren (ed.) *Psychosomatic Medicine. Theory, physiology, and practice*. International Universities Press, Madison, CT.

Watkins, A. (1997) *Mind Body Medicine. A clinician's guide to psychoneuroimmunology*. Churchill Livingstone, New York, Edinburgh, London, Madrid, Melbourne, San Francisco and Tokyo.

Weiner, H. (1977) *Psychobiology and Human Disease*. Elsevier, New York.

Weiner, H. (1989) 'The dynamics of the organism: implications of recent biological thought for psycho-somatic theory and research'. *Psychosomatic Medicine*. 51: 608–35.

Weiner, H. (1991) Stressful experience and cardiorespiratory disorders. *Circulation* 83 11.2–11.8.

Wilding, J. (1997) 'Obesity treatment. A clinical review'. *British Medical Journal* 315: 997–1000.

Wilkie, A. (1993) *Having Cancer and How to Live With It*. Hodder and Stoughton, London.

Williams, R. and Williams, V. (1994) *Anger Kills*. Harper Perennial, London.

Wilson, P. (1999) *The Big Book of Calm. Over 100 successful techniques for relaxing mind and body*. Penguin, London.

Wilson, P. and Mintz, I. (1989) *Psychosomatic Symptoms. Psychodynamic treatment of the underlying personality disorder*. Jason Aronson, Northvale, NJ, London.

Winnicott, D. W. (1947) 'Hate in the countertransference', in *Through Paediatrics to Psycho-Analysis*. Hogarth Press, London, 1975.

Winnicott, D. W.(1964) 'Psycho-somatic illness in its positive and negative aspects', in C. Winnicott, R. Shepherd and M. Davis (eds) *Psycho-Analytic Explorations*. Karnac Books, London, 1989.

Winnicott, D. W. (1969) 'Additional note on psycho-somatic disorder', in C. Winnicott, R. Shepherd and M. Davis (eds) *Psycho-Analytic Explorations*. Karnac Books, London, 1989.

Winnicott, D. W (1971a) *Therapeutic Consultations in Child Psychiatry*. Hogarth Press, London.

Winnicott, D. W. (1971b) *Playing and Reality*. Tavistock Publications, London.

Winnicott, D. W (1972) *The Maturational Processes and the Facilitating Environment*. Hogarth Press, London.

Winnicott, D. W.(1975a) *Through Paediatrics to Psycho-Analysis*. Hogarth Press, London.

Winnicott, D, W. (1975b) 'The observation of infants in a set situation', in *Through Paediatrics to Psycho-Analysis*. Hogarth Press, London.

Winnicott, D. W (1986) 'Cure', in C. Winnicott, R. Shepherd and M. Davis (eds) *Home is Where we Start From. Essays by a psychoanalyst*. Penguin, London.

Winnicott, D. W. (1988) *Human Nature*. Free Association Books, London.

Wolff, H., Bateman, A. and Sturgeon, D. (1990) *UCH Textbook of Psychiatry*. Duckworth, London.

Wurmser, L. (1994) *The Mask of Shame*. Jason Aronson, Northvale, NJ, London.

Zalidis, S. (1991) 'Psychosomatic encounters and the scope for interpretation in general practice'. *Journal of the Balint Society* 19: 16–22.

Zalidis, S. (1992) 'Holding in general practice'. *Journal of the Balint Society* 20: 4–7.

Zalidis, S. (1994a) 'Handling hyperventilation in general practice'. *Journal of the Balint Society* 22: 8–21.

Zalidis S. (1994b) 'The value of emotional awareness', in A. Erskine and D. Judd (eds) *The Imaginative Body. Psychodynamic therapy in health care*. Whurr Publications, London.

Zalidis, S. (1996) 'The human face of general practice'. *Journal of the Balint Society* 24: 25–32

Zalidis, S.(1997) 'So if there is nothing wrong with me, why does it still hurt?', *Journal of the Balint Society* 25: 7–14.

Zalidis, S. (1998a) 'The emotional context preceding the eruption of herpes zoster. Research in progress'. *Journal of the Balint Society* 26: 43–57.

Zalidis, S. (1998b) 'If your eye offends thee pluck it out. Some thoughts on the relationship between eye pain and emotion'. *Psychoanalytic Psychotherapy*. 12(2): 131–40.

Zalidis, S. (1999) 'The empathic holding of the patient's psychosomatic anxiety in the consultation'. *Journal of the Balint Society* 27: 22–8.

INDEX

Compiled by Sue Carlton